300
30 Minute Workouts
for Busy People

Matthew Johnson

Contents

Introduction / Bio

I began working out for the same reasons as everyone at my high school … to perform better at my sport. I played basketball in high school and my dream was to play in college … until I realized that college coaches weren't exactly beating down the doors of 5'10" white guys that are only marginally athletic. College basketball didn't happen, but college did, and just like my peers at that point in my life I primarily worked out to look good at the beach. I'm not convinced that I resembled David Hasselhoff on spring break, but I did build some good habits during that time. In fact, I became a certified personal trainer after my freshman year and worked as the strength and conditioning coach for the Lady Bulldog softball team my junior year. Following college, I spent one misguided year in law school which I made it through 100% due to my daily workout routine. After dropping out of law school, I enrolled in business school and later a graduate exercise science program. While studying exercise science I was exposed to several interesting research projects and helped teach a collegiate strength conditioning class. Following grad school I interned and later was employed at a startup medical clinic/gym, and later became a part owner of a gym. Currently I teach small group HIIT classes and work with individuals one on one. The workouts in this book are the result of the culmination of my years of experience and education in exercise science, strength and conditioning, and personal training. They are intended to simply help everyone from the novice to the most experienced of lifters get a great workout in even when they are extremely busy.

What this book is not

This book is not a workout program. This book is also not a novel, meaning that it is not intended for you to read from cover to cover, although feel free to if you wish. This book does contain "beginner" workouts, although it is not necessarily for beginners. This book is not a step-by-step guide to losing weight or building muscle, even though it does include a great deal of information that will help you do both of those things. This book is not going to provide illustrations on how to complete many exercises, although it does provide some written explanation on how to perform some exercises.

What this book is

This book is a collection of 300 workouts that can be completed on any given day very quickly. The book is organized first based on the body part(s) that you are working on a given day and secondly by the type of muscular development that you are trying to achieve. For example, if you are working your way through a strength building workout program and your program calls for you to complete a strength workout that focuses primarily on shoulder exercises, but you don't have time to complete a long shoulder workout, you could pick up this book and just flip to the shoulder chapter and find the strength section to insert a one-day, 30 minute shoulder strength workout. Additionally, if you're like me and you become increasingly bored with long workout programs and like to freestyle your workouts based on how you feel that day, this book is an excellent resource to use if you don't quite know what you want to do in the gym on a given day. This book is more like a recipe book than a workout program in that it will list all of the ingredients and show you how to put the workout together, but it will not develop a meal plan for you. I am all for workout plans, and I believe that most people can benefit from some of the great plans out there. However, I also know that most people do not stick with these plans and are more likely to wing it in the gym every day. Consider this book a safer alternative to winging it.

Disclaimer

The exercises in this book are organized as "Beginner," "Intermediate," and "Advanced." Although I did my best to tailor the beginner workouts to the needs of true beginners, I strongly recommend meeting with a certified personal trainer to complete a fitness assessment before trying these workouts. If you have a pre-existing metabolic condition you need to seek clearance from a medical doctor before starting to exercise. If you have a pre-existing issue that impacts your mobility I recommend meeting with a physical or occupational therapist prior to beginning to exercise. There are a number of free resources available online that demonstrate how to correctly perform the exercises in the book. Examples of many, but not all of these exercises can be found on 300quickworkouts.com. I encourage you to push yourself, but do so within reason. The workouts in this book were developed based on a combination of the fitness and strength training research, experience with my clients, and my own trial and error. I do not guarantee that these workouts are safe and effective for everyone, but I have made every effort for them to be.

Big Thanks

First, big thanks to my wife, Anna for supporting this big idea and the late/early hours it took to develop 300 workouts. Big thanks to my parents and sister for their ongoing support. Big thanks to Davie for his superb editing skills. Big Thanks to Roger and Franklin for their stellar pseudo-legal advice. Big thanks to Pam for the awesome cover. Big thanks to Tyler, Brandon, Chris, and Matt, who all indicated that this was a good idea. And big thanks to anyone else who has supported this project in any way, including those who purchased the book!

Glossary / Terms

To be able to effectively use this book you will need to understand some fairly basic definitions. These definitions are far from all encompassing, but they will help you understand how this book is organized and how to use it effectively.

Definitions:

- **Class:** Each workout table contains a "Class" section that will indicate which training range this workout falls under. This is primarily determined by the number of sets and reps in the workout, however, other factors such as rest period duration, load (resistance), and whether other intensity implements such as super-sets are used in the workout. While each workout will lean toward a single class, they will all bleed into each other to some degree. Most strength workouts will help develop some power and build some muscle, just as most power workouts will help to develop strength. These are not set in stone; they are a simple guide-line.

- **Power**
  - **Definition(s):** Power is the rate at which work is completed. Further, work is the product of the force exerted on an object and the distance that object moves in the direction in which the force is exerted (8).

  - **Example:** A measurement of power would be the rate at which a bench press is completed relative to the weight that is being lifted.

  - **Purpose:** The purpose of developing power is quite simple: aspects of every sport, as well as many "real life" situations, require a certain degree of power to complete at a high level. Further, in most situations having more power is a competitive advantage that can help lead to success in the task. Lastly, performing exercises in a way that develops power typically stimulates fast twitch muscle fibers, which can help lead to greater hypertrophy gains, as fast twitch fibers have relatively more potential for growth than do their slow twitch counterparts (11).

- **Strength**

    o **Definition(s):** The maximal force that a muscle or muscle group can generate at a specific velocity (8).

    o **Example:** The maximum bench press test. Here, an individual attempts to measure the strength of the upper body and particularly of the chest, shoulders, and triceps muscles by lifting the most weight that they can lift for one rep of the bench press exercise.

    o **Purpose:** Just as with power development, greater levels of strength can help improve performance in both athletics and daily activities.

- **Hypertrophy**

    o **Definition(s):** Hypertrophy refers to the increase in muscle cell size as a result of resistance training. Specifically, the term refers to an increase in actin and myosin filaments that comprise a great majority of the cross sectional area of a muscle fiber. Although hypertrophy is not technically the only way that muscle grows (hyperplasia, actually growing new muscle cells, may take place to a small extent), the term "Hypertrophy" will be used interchangeably with "Muscle Growth" throughout this book (11).

    o **Example:** The increase in upper-arm circumference after an 8 week resistance training program that includes consistent stimulus to the biceps muscles.

    o **Purpose:** Everyone wants to gain muscle. Some people say that they want to "tone" a muscle, rather than to gain muscle, but toning a muscle is merely a myth. In order to improve your body's "tone" or definition, you simply need to lose body fat and build muscle. This is where hypertrophy becomes so important.

- **Muscular Endurance**

  - **Definition(s):** Muscular endurance refers to a muscle's ability to contract against a given resistance over a period of time (9).

  - **Example:** Look at an Olympic rower's back muscles, specifically the latissimus dorsi. Those muscles must continually contract throughout a competition against a fairly consistent resistance. A rower who has higher local muscular endurance will be able to row at a given pace over a longer period of time than a rower with lower muscular endurance.

  - **Purpose:** It is important to develop muscular endurance in order to be able to perform at a high level over a longer time period. Power, strength, and muscle hypertrophy are all very important, but it is also important to be able to use those over a fairly long period of time without fatiguing.

- **Level**

  - **Definition(s):** In this book, the level of the workout simply refers to how experienced a person needs to be to complete the workout relative to the intensity of the workout. Which "Level" you are is determined by you, but typically a beginner is anyone with less than one year of consistent strength training and conditioning experience, a person is intermediate if they have 1 – 3 years of experience training, and a person is advanced if they have greater than 3 years of experience. However, even though you may not fall into the advanced category you can still complete most of the advanced workouts by scaling them to your level.

  - **Example:** If you are an intermediate lifter, scaling a workout to your level would be to complete a workout using straight sets instead of super-sets, if the workout calls for super-sets. Another way to scale is to simply cut out some of the more difficult exercises that you are not familiar with, such as power cleans, hang-cleans, bent rows, or squats. Exercises such as those require a high degree of technicality and need to be taught by a professional with a great deal of experience and education in strength and conditioning.

- o **Purpose:** Although we all have different strengths and weaknesses, it is important to provide a reference point for how difficult each workout will be and who each workout is generally intended for.

- **Time**

  - o **Definition(s):** The time category simply provides an estimate for how long it will take to complete each workout. This does not include warm-up or cool down sessions, so be sure to factor those in.

  - o **Example:** Don't schedule an important meeting after a workout just because it claims to take only 20 minutes … it may take you 30.

  - o **Purpose:** Time estimates are provided for each workout in order to hold you accountable to staying on task, implementing necessary rest between sets, and ensuring that desired intensity levels are being achieved.

- **Resistance (%1RM)**

  - o **Definition(s):** The resistance category in the table provides a general guideline to the amount of resistance that you will need to use in order for the given exercise or set to be effective. Most of the workouts will feature the word "Resistance (%)." The % is referring to the %1RM for the given lift. %1 RM is the percentage of your one rep max on a given lift. This is the amount of weight that you could lift for one repetition on an exercise. Keep in mind that this is simply a guideline or starting point to help you figure out how much resistance to use. There will still be a great deal of trial and error when figuring the correct weight, so keep that in mind and don't get too caught up trying to figure the exact %1RM for each exercise (9).

- Example: If your 1RM on the bench press is 200 pounds, then you can bench press 200 pounds one time, and no more than one time in a single set. So if a workout calls for you to complete 15 reps at 50% of your 1RM, you should use 100 pounds to complete the 15 reps. There are several ways to measure or estimate 1RM, ranging from a direct max bench press test to other indirect tests that include formulas to estimate 1RM (9).

- Purpose: For the purpose of this book, %1RM is meant to be an estimate of the intensity that you will need on a given exercise. Testing for 1RM is generally safe, so long as you have the proper equipment, resources, and personnel. Testing your 1RM on each exercise is not necessary in order to use this book. Rather, the %1RM is meant to guide you to a weight that allows you to complete the prescribed number of sets and reps, but no more than the prescribed number of sets and reps. For instance, if a workout calls for three sets of 10 bench presses with 65% of your 1RM for the intensity, you should be able to estimate how much weight on the bar would allow you to complete three sets of 10 with good form, while staying within an 8 to 12 rep range.

- **Rest Periods**

  - The bottom of each workout table spells out the prescribed rest periods for each workout. These rest periods refer to the rest that is recommended between each set. Again, like the prescribed resistance, rest needs will vary from person to person and may require some trial and error to get right. Feel free to time your rest periods with precision if you wish, but that may not be necessary. Just be cognizant of how long you are resting and try not to sit around and talk for 3 minutes between sets if the workout calls for only 20 seconds of rest.

- **Muscle Fiber Types**

  o There are several references to muscle fiber types throughout this book, most of which focus on which type of muscle fibers mostly correlate with the exercise being performed. There are two key differentiating factors in muscle fiber types; contractile properties and metabolic properties.

  - **Type 1 Muscle Fiber**

    • These muscle fibers, commonly referred to as slow twitch muscle fibers, have nearly half of the contractile components that type 2, or fast twitch muscle fibers have, doubling their time to peak tension compared to fast twitch fibers. Conversely, type 1 fibers are comprised of more mitochondria and have a higher capillary density than type 2 fibers, meaning that they can contract for a much longer period of time (11).

    • Workouts in the endurance sections of the book, as well as some of the mixed workouts, will primarily target type 1 muscle fibers because the duration of the sets will dictate that these muscle cells continue to contract when the type 2 cells have long stopped. Aerobic exercise primarily targets type 1 muscle fibers.

  - **Type 2 Muscle Fiber**

    • Type 2 muscle fibers have twice as much surface area of key contractile components, making contraction stronger and time to peak tension shorter. This allows for a much stronger muscle contraction, but one that can last for only a short period of time. Anaerobic workouts in the power and strength sections of the book will typically target fast twitch muscle fibers (11).

Quick Terms

- **AMAP:** As Many As Possible
- **Intensity:** The relative difficulty of a workout as a result of the combination of sets, reps, resistance, and rest period length.
- **Concentric Portion:** This is the exertive portion of a lift. Example: the push phase of a bench press exercise.
- **Eccentric Portion:** This is the "passive" portion of a lift. Example: The lowering down phase of a bench press exercise.
- **Rep(s):** Short for repetitions. Each time you complete the concentric and eccentric portion of an exercise you have completed one rep.
- **Set:** A group or series of exercises with a prescribed number of reps that are completed before moving onto the next exercise. For example, if a workout calls for three sets of 10 reps on the chest press machine, you would complete 10 reps, rest, complete another 10 reps, rest, and then complete the last "set" of 10 reps before moving onto the next exercise.
- **Super-set:** A super-set is the combination of a set of two different exercises without rest. For example, if a workout calls for a super-set of 10 reps of push-ups and 10 reps of pull-ups, you would complete 10 push-ups followed immediately by 10 pull-ups without rest. You would rest after the completion of the second exercise in the super-set.
- **Giant Set:** This is also considered a double super-set, where you complete sets of three different exercises in a row without rest.
- **Lb.** Pound
- **Lbs.** Pounds
- **Pin Drop:** This simply refers to the style of resistance machine that uses a pin to select the weight that you want to use.
- **Protagonist Muscles:** Muscles that are the prime movers in an exercise.
- **Antagonist Muscles:** Muscles that are in direct opposition to the prime movers of an exercise.
- **Stabilizers:** Muscles that are not the protagonist or antagonist muscles in an exercise but still work to keep the body in optimal position during the exercise. Very often the muscles of the core.
- **BW:** Body Weight resistance.
- **Unilateral:** One side at a time.
- **Functional Training:** Training that more resembles daily activity. Most exercises involve a relatively greater amount of

movement and require more balance and stabilization than other exercises.

- **Spotter:** Someone standing (mostly) behind you during a lift who is prepared to help you safely lift the weight in the event that you fail to complete a rep.
- **Straight Set:** A set of repetitions that is followed by a rest period.

Chapter 1

Chest Workouts

If you're like me, you believe that chest day truly is the best day. When I think of weight lifting, the first exercise that comes to mind is the bench press. The bench press is the king of upper-body exercises because it allows you to work a large number of muscle groups, including the chest, shoulders and triceps directly. Additionally, the bench press allows you to lift more weight than any other strictly upper body move, making it ideal for helping you to boost both size and strength. Many people begin their week with chest day because it is simply their favorite or because they believe that their chest needs the most improvement and therefore needs to be worked when they are most rested. Regardless of why or when you work your chest, insert a workout from this chapter to help you achieve your targeted results. Keep in mind that a later chapter will feature workouts for both chest and triceps work as well as chest and back; moreover, if you have longer than 30 minutes to complete a workout, feel free to add a triceps, back, biceps, or core workout on to the end of the chest workout that you choose. Also keep in mind that the time allocation for each workout does not include time for warming up. However, almost all of these workouts can be completed in 30 minutes or less including warmup time. A good warmup for the chest workouts would involve a light-weight, high rep scheme such as a series of push-ups or bench presses with light weight on the bar.

Chest: Power Workouts

Workout 1
Chest Day Best Day

Class	Difficulty Level	Time
Power	Beginner	30 minutes

This workout is meant to help you develop power, not only in your chest, but throughout your entire body. The key here is to go heavy enough to justify performing so few reps, but light enough to be able to develop a high velocity during the lift. Though this may not look like a great amount of volume, training for power requires the use of both an appropriate amount of weight and rest throughout the workout.

Exercise	Sets	Reps	Resistance (%)
Flat Plate Loaded Press	3	3	75-85
Dumbbell Bench Press	3	4	75-85
Cable Crossover	3	5	75-85
Rest Periods	2 minutes		

Workout 2
Power Bench

Class	Difficulty Level	Time
Power	Beginner	30 minutes

Here, we are sticking to the pin drop bench press 100%. This is a convenient workout if you are a beginner or if you don't have a spotter. If you decide to complete this workout in consecutive weeks, try to increase the weight used by 3 - 5% each week. Remember, your body has to respond to the increased stress that you are putting on it by becoming stronger and more powerful.

Exercise	Sets	Reps	Resistance (%)
Pin Drop Chest Press	5	3	60,70,80,70, 60
Rest Periods	3 minutes		

Workout 3
Rise of the Chest Machines

Class	Difficulty Level	Time
Power	Intermediate	30 minutes

The great thing about this workout is that you don't need to worry about having a spotter to complete it safely. What you do need, however, is a gym that happens to have several variations of the plate-loaded chest-press machine. Although there is no great substitute for free-weight lifting, it doesn't hurt to mix things up every once in a while to break past a plateau or to give certain muscle groups (particularly stabilizers) a rest while concentrating on others.

Exercise	Sets	Reps	Resistance (%)
Plate Loaded Flat Press	3	3 - 4	75
Plate Loaded Incline Press	3	3 - 4	75
Flat Plate Loaded Decline Press	3	3 - 4	75
Rest Periods	2 minutes		

Workout 4
Plyo Chest

Class	Difficulty Level	Time
Power	Intermediate	25 minutes

Just because you want to be more powerful doesn't mean that you can't throw some bodyweight or lighter weight stuff into the mix. Here, your goal is to teach your body to perform the concentric portions of these exercises as quickly as possible after performing the eccentric portions at a normal pace. This may not sound all that difficult, but after performing the lifts as quickly as possible you will likely be pretty exhausted.

Exercise	Sets	Reps	Resistance (%)
Flat Bench Press	4	4	50
Clap Pushup	5	5	BW
Rest Periods	2 minutes		

Workout 5
Power Smith

Class	Difficulty Level	Time
Power	Advanced	25 minutes

Although Smith Machines should probably not be relied on exclusively, they are good to incorporate into a routine if you work out alone, are trying to break through a plateau, or are simply getting bored with your normal workouts. Because the weight is on tracks, you do not have to expend much energy stabilizing the movement, but you still need to be careful, as you can get trapped under the bar if it is between safety hooks when you fail on a lift. After the four heavy sets, perform five sets at 30-50% of your one rep max (1RM). Perform these reps as explosively as possible, and if you have a spotter, you can even try releasing the bar at the top of the concentric portion of the lift and then catching the bar on the way down.

Exercise	Sets	Reps	Resistance (%)
Flat Smith Press	4	4	75-85
Flat Smith Press	5	5	30-50
Rest Periods	2 minutes		

Workout 6
Power Cable Workout

Class	Difficulty Level	Time
Power	Advanced	20 minutes

This workout only requires a corner cable crossover machine, sometimes referred to as a functional trainer. These machines are typically more suited for strength, hypertrophy, or endurance workouts because they bring stabilizer muscles into play to a high degree. However, if you are working out in a hotel or some other facility that lacks a wide variety of equipment you can still gain some power with this workout. Perform both sets of the cable crosses and push-ups as supersets to add intensity to this workout.

Exercise	Sets	Reps	Resistance (%)
Standing Cable Press	4	5	85
Clap Push-up	4	5	BW
Standing Cable Cross	3	8	80
Push-up	3	8	BW
Rest Periods	90 seconds		

Chest: Strength Workouts

Workout 7
Arnold

Class	Difficulty Level	Time
Strength	Beginner	30 minutes

This workout is meant to help you work on your strength, but the rep range and volume will certainly bleed into hypertrophy training as well. Notice that the bench press and dumbbell bench press tend to come first in these workouts; this is because they both require a great amount of stabilization from other muscles, unlike the machine exercises.

Exercise	Sets	Reps	Resistance (%)
Bench Press	2	6 - 8	75
Dumbbell Bench Press	2	6 - 8	75
Incline Plate Loaded	2	8 - 10	75
Decline Plate Loaded	2	8 – 10	75
Rest Periods		90 – 120 seconds	

Workout 8
Functional Strength

Class	Difficulty Level	Time
Strength	Beginner	25 minutes

This workout is for beginners looking to add upper body strength. To perform incline push-ups, place your feet on a 12 – 18 inch plyo box or flat bench and bend over with your palms touching the floor in a push-up position. To perform decline push-ups, do just the opposite… place the palms of your hands on flat bench in a push-up position. Using different angles on any exercise will help to target both different muscles and different parts of particular muscles (2), which is why incline and decline push-ups are recommended here. Remember to keep your back flat and chest up on all of these exercises.

Exercise	Sets	Reps	Resistance
Push-ups	3	6 - 8	BW
TRX Chest Press	3	6 - 8	BW
Incline Push-ups	3	6 - 8	BW
Decline Push-ups	3	6 – 8	BW
Rest Periods		90 seconds	

Workout 9
The Machine Master

Class	Difficulty Level	Time
Strength	Intermediate	30 minutes

Like the power chest machine workout, this workout allows you to improve your strength if you do not have a spotter, need to break through a plateau, or are becoming tired of your typical free-weight routine. To mix this up a bit, perform the second set of each exercise unilaterally, holding the press at the top portion while your other arm presses up. For example, on flat chest press start by pressing with your right arm only and, while holding the weight at the top press with your left hand. Once your left side is up, let the right down and press it back up immediately.

Exercise	Sets	Reps	Resistance (%)
Flat Plate Loaded	2	6 - 8	75
Wide Plate Loaded	2	6 - 8	75
Incline Plate Loaded	2	6 - 8	75
Decline Plate Loaded	2	6 – 8	75
Rest Periods		90 seconds – 2 minutes	

Workout 10
Dumbbell Heyday

Class	Difficulty Level	Time
Strength	Intermediate	30 minutes

This workout is difficult because of the degree of stabilization that takes place when you use dumbbells. However, this should help you to bust through strength plateaus and reach new levels of strength on all of your lifts. If you have longer than 30 minutes, you could increase the number of sets to three each in order to significantly increase the volume completed.

Exercise	Sets	Reps	Resistance (%)
Flat Dumbbell Press	2	6 - 8	80 - 85
Incline Dumbbell Press	2	6 - 8	80 - 85
Decline Dumbbell Press	2	6 - 8	80 - 85
Flat Dumbbell Fly	2	6 – 8	80 - 85
Rest Periods		90 seconds	

Workout 11
Smith Strength

Class	Difficulty Level	Time
Strength	Advanced	30 minutes

The goal in incorporating rest-pause training is to be able to lift a given weight for more volume than you would be able to in a straight set (7). Here, pick a weight that you could only perform 4 repetitions with. Complete 3 reps, rest 15 – 20 seconds, and then explosively complete 2 – 3 more reps. Do this for each exercise, except for the last, where you will be performing one arm presses.

Exercise	Sets	Reps	Resistance (%)
Flat Smith Press	2	3 + 3	70 - 80
Incline Smith Press	2	3 + 3	70 - 80
Decline Smith Press	2	3 + 3	70 - 80
Flat Unilateral Press	2	5 (each side)	70 – 80
Rest Periods			90 seconds

Workout 12
From the Bottom

Class	Difficulty Level	Time
Strength	Advanced	30 minutes

Place a flat bench inside a lifting cage and move the safety bars on the sides so that they are parallel with 1 – 2 inches above your chest when you lay flat. Place a barbell on the safeties and lay down underneath it in a bench press position. Check to make sure that the safeties are high enough, and then load the bar with your ten rep max weight. Lay back in a bench press position and bench press the bar as you normally would. Lower the bar back down to the safeties and let it rest for 2 seconds before completing your next rep. Concentric-only training is intended to prevent your muscles from being able to use the stored energy in the muscle fibers immediately following an eccentric load, forcing your muscles to rely only on the concentric portion of the subsequent lift and therefore strengthening that portion of the lift (3, 4, 5).

Exercise	Sets	Reps	Resistance (%)
Flat Bench Press	5	6	80 - 85
Rest Periods			90 seconds

Chest: Muscle Building Workouts

Class	Difficulty Level	Time
Muscle Building	Beginner	25 minutes

This is a very straightforward workout. Load the bench with 65 – 75% of your 1RM and complete ten sets of 10 bench presses. This workout saves time by keeping you from having to jump around from station to station changing weight and waiting on someone to get out of your way. Try to use the same weight throughout the workout, but if you need to reduce the weight on the last set or two, there's no shame in that game.

Exercise	Sets	Reps	Resistance (%)
Flat Bench Press	10	10	65 - 75
Rest Periods	90 seconds		

Workout 14
Push it Up

Class	Difficulty Level	Time
Muscle Building	Beginner	25 minutes

This workout is for beginners, people in a bind without a gym, or anyone who wants to add some functional training to another routine. All you need to complete this workout is you and a chair. If you cannot complete clap push-ups, don't worry; simply perform the push-up as explosively as you can. Complete this workout as a circuit, taking little to no rest between each set except for after completing the last exercise in the circuit.

Exercise	Sets	Reps	Resistance
Clap Push-up	4	5	BW
Incline Push-up	4	5	BW
Decline Push-up	4	5	BW
Normal Push-up	4	5	BW
Rest Periods	2 minutes between circuit		

Workout 15
The Change-up

Class	Difficulty Level	Time
Muscle Building	Intermediate	20 minutes

The most tedious part of this workout is the setup; grab a pair of heavy dumbbells and a pair of light dumbbells, and take them over to a bench press. Load the bench with 50% of your one rep max. Begin by performing 5 regular dumbbell presses with the heavy dumbbells. Without resting, perform 5 regular dumbbell fly's with the lighter dumbbells. Next, again without resting, perform 5 bench presses, moving slowly on the eccentric portion and exploding up on the concentric portion. This workout incorporates supersets, drop sets, and pre-exhaustion all in one working set. Complete 3 – 4 rounds of this and you're finished.

Exercise	Sets	Reps	Resistance (%)
Flat Dumbbell Press	3 - 4	5	80
Flat Dumbbell Fly	3 - 4	5	70
Flat Bench Press	3 - 4	5	50
Rest Periods		2 minutes between circuit	

Workout 16
Drop It likes It's HUGE

Class	Difficulty Level	Time
Muscle Building	Intermediate	30 minutes

This workout introduces drop sets as a way to increase intensity. To perform drop sets, start with a weight that you can only perform 6 – 8 reps with, complete those reps, and then drop the weight by around 20% and immediately complete 4 – 6 more reps. Training this way may help you to recruit additional muscle fibers once you fail on the first portion of the set, effectively helping your muscle building efforts (10).

Exercise	Sets	Reps	Resistance (%)
Flat Dumbbell Press	2	6 + 4	85 + 65
Incline Dumbbell Press	2	6 + 4	85 + 65
Decline Smith Press	2	6 + 4	85 + 65
Cable Crossover	2	6 + 4	85 + 65
Rest Periods		60 seconds	

9

Workout 17
If You're So Inclined

Class	Difficulty Level	Time
Muscle Building	Advanced	30 minutes

Here, you will use supersets between incline dumbbell presses and incline dumbbell fly's, as well as between incline push-ups and incline cable crossovers. This workout is meant to target the upper portion of your chest and will also impact your shoulders, particularly your front deltoids, to a large degree.

Exercise	Sets	Reps	Resistance (%)
Incline Dumbbell Press	2	10	75
Incline Dumbbell Fly	2	10	75
Incline Push-ups	2	10	75
Incline Cable Crossover	2	10	75
Rest Periods			60 seconds

Workout 18
Decline Dominate

Class	Difficulty Level	Time
Muscle Building	Advanced	30 minutes

If you're trying to develop your lower chest area, try this workout. This workout hits the lower chest with a variety of moves and can be completed fairly quickly with the use of super sets. Here, complete the decline dumbbell presses and the decline dumbbell fly's back to back with no rest. Do the same with the weighted dips and the cable crossovers.

Exercise	Sets	Reps	Resistance (%)
Decline Dumbbell Press	2	10	75
Decline Dumbbell Fly	2	10	75
Weighted Dips	2	10	75
Cable Crossover	2	10	75
Rest Periods			60 seconds

Chest: Endurance Workouts

Workout 19
Push-up Marathon

Class	Difficulty Level	Time
Endurance	Beginner	12 minutes

This workout challenges the endurance levels of the muscles in your chest, triceps, and front deltoids. Here, complete 50 push-ups in as many sets as it takes to get to 50. For example, you might perform a set of 20 pushups, rest, then complete a set of 15 push-ups, rest, then complete subsequent sets of 10 and 5. Take only as much rest as absolutely necessary between sets, as this workout is meant to push your muscles to your lactate threshold. Once you can perform 50 push-ups in one set, complete the same workout for 100 push-ups.

Exercise	Sets	Reps	Resistance
Flat Push-up	1 - 12	50	BW
Rest Periods	20 seconds between sets		

Workout 20
½ Bodyweight Bench Press

Class	Difficulty Level	Time
Endurance	Intermediate	20 minutes

This workout simply seeks to determine how many times you can bench press half of your bodyweight. First, weigh yourself to determine your weight. Next, load the bar with half of that amount. For example, if you weigh 200 pounds, load the bar with 100 pounds. Complete five sets to failure, but make sure you have a spotter on this one. The amount of reps that a person can complete on this exercise will vary a great deal from person to person, as everyone is different in terms of muscular strength and size, fat mass, height, and so on.

Exercise	Sets	Reps	Resistance (%)
Flat Bench Press	5	AMAP	½ BW
Rest Periods	2 minutes between sets		

Workout 21
Bottom to Top Cable Cross

Class	Difficulty Level	Time
Endurance	Intermediate	20 minutes

There comes a time in every gym-goer's experience that they just need a break from pressing... this is it. If you feel over-fatigued and your joints are aching, but you still want to get a good chest workout in, you've come to the right place. Stand inside a cable machine with the cables on each side placed on the bottom selection. Perform incline cable crosses, bringing the cables from down to your sides to crossing up to parallel with your chin. Complete 10 reps, then bend down and raise each cable attachment up two slots and repeat. Continue this process until you have completed decline cable crossovers from the top setting on each side of the crossover machine.

Exercise	Sets	Reps	Resistance (%)
Cable Crossover	10	10	60 - 70
Rest Periods		15 seconds between sets	

Workout 22
Chest Press Pin Drop

Class	Difficulty Level	Time
Endurance	Intermediate	15 minutes

This workout is very simple. Sit in a chest press machine that features a pin-select mechanism to increase or decrease the weighted resistance. Place the pin on your 2 rep max, and complete 2 reps. Immediately pull the pin up and place it on the next lightest weight. Complete 4 reps, and continue this exercise until you have reached the lightest weight and are completing around 20 reps. The advantage of performing a drop set to increase endurance over simply one light set is that you are pushing against adequate resistance as your muscle fatigues, rather than the set being very easy at the beginning and difficult at the end with a light weight.

Exercise	Sets	Reps	Resistance
Flat Pin – Select press	6 - 8	2,4,6,8,10,12,14,16,18,20	Varies
Rest Periods		10 seconds between sets	

Workout 23
Triple Dipping

Class	Difficulty Level	Time
Endurance	Advanced	15 minutes

In this workout you want to test the strength of the lower chest, shoulders and triceps over an extended period of time. To do this, grab a lifting belt, a chain, and either a 10 or 20 pound weight plate. Attach the weight plate to the chain, and the chain to the lifting belt, and then perform 5 dips. After these 5, immediately remove the weight belt, and complete 5 explosive dips, which means that you will lower yourself under control, explode upwards, rest and repeat. After completing 5 reps, immediately complete 5 normal dips. Remember to keep your back flat and your chest up, with your legs kicked back behind you to emphasize the chest muscles in this workout. Do not try this workout if you cannot complete 10 normal dips, 10 weighted dips, or 10 explosive dips in straight sets.

Exercise	Sets	Reps	Resistance
Weighted Dips	3	5	10 – 25 lbs.
Plyo Dips	3	5	BW
Normal Dips	3	5	BW
Rest Periods		2 minutes between sets	

Workout 24
Running the Rack

Class	Difficulty Level	Time
Endurance	Advanced	15 minutes

Here, pick a weight that is 90% of your 1RM and complete 4 reps of flat dumbbell press. Immediately rack the weight and grab the pair of dumbbells that are 10 pounds lighter and complete 6 reps. Repeat until you reach 20 reps. At this point, rest for 2 minutes and repeat the entire process, only this time begin with the weight that you used for your second set in the first round.

Exercise	Sets	Reps	Resistance
Flat Dumbbell Press	6 – 8 (3 rounds)	4,6,8,10,12,14,16,18,20	Varies
Rest Periods		5 minutes between rounds	

Chest: Mixed Workouts

Workout 25
Bench Pyramid

Class	Difficulty Level	Time
Mixed	Beginner	30 minutes

Pyramids are a great way to work on power, strength, hypertrophy and endurance all in the same workout. Begin this bench press sequence with 65% of your 1RM and complete 10 reps. Next, add 10 pounds to each side and complete 8 reps. Subsequently add 10 more pounds to each side and complete 8 reps. Continue this trend down to 6 reps and then begin pyramiding back up and stop at 10 reps. This workout can also be done with dumbbells, a plate-loaded machine, or a pin-select machine if you don't have a spotter.

Exercise	Sets	Reps	Resistance (%)
Bench Press	5	10,8,6,8,10	Varies
Rest Periods		90 seconds between sets	

Workout 26
Push-Fly

Class	Difficulty Level	Time
Mixed	Intermediate	30 minutes

In this workout, you will simply perform a dumbbell press followed by a dumbbell fly. This workout is fairly straightforward and can probably be completed in 20 minutes, as there is very minimal setup. If you do want to add an extra element of endurance and added intensity to the workout, you could perform flat, incline, and decline push-ups following the completion of each set of fly's.

Exercise	Sets	Reps	Resistance (%)
Flat Dumbbell Press	2	6 - 8	70 - 80
Flat Dumbbell Fly	2	6 - 8	70 - 80
Incline Dumbbell Press	2	6 - 8	70 - 80
Incline Dumbbell Fly	2	6 - 8	70 - 80
Decline Dumbbell Press	2	6 - 8	70 - 80
Decline Dumbbell Fly	2	6 - 8	70 - 80
Rest Periods		90 seconds between sets	

Workout 27
The Athlete

Class	Difficulty Level	Time
Mixed	Intermediate	30 minutes

This workout focuses on strength and hypertrophy by incorporating more exercises that bring stabilizing muscles into play. First, complete 8 flat dumbbell presses with each arm, one at a time by holding the first press at the top portion while your other arm presses up. Start by performing a chest press with only your right arm, hold at the finishing portion of the lift, and press up with your left to meet it at the top. Once your left side is up, lower the right down and press it back up immediately. Upon finishing the first exercise, load 50% of your 1RM on the bench press and complete four sets of 4 reps, lowering the weight slowly and under control and then explosively pressing it up again. This workout is meant to help you gain strength and increase muscle while also activating your stabilizer muscles.

Exercise	Sets	Reps	Resistance (%)
Flat Unilateral Dumbbell press	4	8	65 - 75
Flat Bench Press	4	4	50
Rest Periods		90 seconds between sets	

Workout 28
Stair-Step Chest

Class	Difficulty Level	Time
Mixed	Intermediate	30 minutes

This workout, as with all of the mixed workouts, is meant to borrow set, rep and weight schemes from the power, strength, muscle building, and endurance workouts. Here, begin the workout with low volume, high weight, and long rest periods, and end it with high volume, low weight, and short rest periods. Give your chest a week to recover from this workout … it will need it.

Exercise	Sets	Reps	Resistance (%)
Bench Press	2	4	85 - 90
Incline Dumbbell Press	3	8	70 - 80
Decline Dumbbell Press	3	8	70 - 80
Flat Dumbbell Fly	Run the rack	10	70 - 30
Rest Periods		2 minutes between sets	

Workout 29
Mega Chest

Class	Difficulty Level	Time
Mixed	Advanced	30 minutes

To complete this workout, place an incline bench press inside of a cable crossover machine. Place the cables at the bottom of the machine, and select a weight that you can complete for 10 reps. Next, grab a pair of dumbbells that weigh around 85% of your 1RM and place them at the foot of the bench. Now, if your gym has fixed barbells, grab one that weighs around 50% of your 1RM and place it in front of the dumbbells on the floor. Now you're ready to start the workout. Begin by completing 10 dumbbell presses. Once you complete 10, immediately drop the dumbbells to the side and grab the cables. Complete 10 incline cable crossovers then drop the cables and pick up the fixed barbell. Complete 10 incline barbell presses and put the barbell down (this can be tricky, so be careful) and rest.

Exercise	Sets	Reps	Resistance (%)
Incline Dumbbell Press	3	4	85
Incline Cable Crossover	3	8	70
Incline Barbell Press	3	8	50
Rest Periods		2 minutes between sets	

Workout 30
Forced Rep Chest

Class	Difficulty Level	Time
Mixed	Advanced	30 minutes

Here, perform dumbbell bench presses taking two seconds to press the weight up and four seconds to lower the weight back down. At failure, have your spotter help you complete however many more reps that you need to get to 10. However, if you do not complete at least 5 reps, lower the weight by at least 10 pounds prior to the next set. The goal here is to pick a weight that causes you to fail at between 6 and 8 reps.

Exercise	Sets	Reps	Resistance (%)
Flat Dumbbell Press	3	6 + 4	80
Incline Dumbbell Press	3	6 + 4	80
Decline Dumbbell Press	3	6 + 4	80
Rest Periods		90 seconds between sets	

16

Chapter 2

Back Workouts

Working on the chest, biceps, shoulders and abs is very popular because these are the muscles that we see in the mirror. However, it's equally important to concentrate on the muscles in your back. Developing these muscles will prevent imbalances in strength and musculature that could cause you to become more susceptible to injury (2, 10). While it is important to develop power in the back muscles, it is impossible to do so in a vacuum, as other muscles will come into play to a large degree. Rather than thinking of the power workouts in this chapter as developing power in the back alone, think of them more in terms of developing power throughout the entire body. For example, one of the best exercises to develop power in the back muscles is the deadlift, which many would consider a leg exercise. Because of this, you will notice the deadlift can be found in both the back and leg section, which is normal. Additionally, the muscles of the trapezius are part of the back musculature but are often worked with shoulders instead. Because of this, there will also be some overlap between shoulders and back with exercises like the shrug, power clean and hang clean. Another caveat to consider with back training is that many of the muscles in the back, particularly the postural muscles of the lower back, are comprised of a greater amount of slow-twitch muscle fibers that are meant to contract over long periods of time. As a result, it is important to continue to train the lower back muscles for strength and endurance even when you are trying to develop power. Speaking of lower back muscles, keep in mind that warming up before performing deadlifts and other back exercises is crucial. While the estimated exercise times listed do not include time for a warmup, almost all of these workouts can still be completed in 30 minutes even after you warm up. A good warmup for back exercises would be a series of dynamic exercises that target the muscles of the middle, outer and lower back as well as the biceps. Completing a series of light cable rows or lat pull-downs is advised.

Back: Power Workouts

Workout 31
Back Machine Day

Class	Difficulty Level	Time
Power	Beginner	25 minutes

Here, you can give your stabilizers a bit of break and load up the back row machines to develop power in the back. This is a good option if you have already worked your legs hard this week and need to give them a break.

Exercise	Sets	Reps	Resistance (%)
Plate Loaded Row	4	4	70-80
Plate Loaded Pull-down	4	4	70-80
Rest Periods		90 seconds between sets	

Workout 32
Dead Shrug

Class	Difficulty Level	Time
Power	Beginner	20 minutes

This workout can be completed quickly, as there is very little in the way of setup. Here, perform five sets of 4 deadlifts with 2 shrugs on the top of each rep. This will help to develop the muscles from bottom to top in the back, ranging from the postural muscles in the lower back, the trapezius and rhomboids in the middle back, and the latissimus dorsi muscles on the outer parts of the back.

Exercise	Sets	Reps	Resistance (%)
Shrug Plus	5	4 + 2	65
Rest Periods		90 seconds between sets	

Workout 33
Heavy Pull-Ups

Class	Difficulty Level	Time
Power	Intermediate	30 minutes

This workout is primarily meant to challenge and develop your lats, but most of the muscles in your body will contribute in one way or another. Begin by performing one of the most challenging and explosive movements in the gym: an explosive pull-up. The goal is to pull yourself up as explosively as you can, let your hands leave the bar as you approach the top portion of the pull-up, and then return to the bar on your way back down. Gravity makes performing this exercise especially challenging, so make sure that you are able to do several weighted pull-ups before attempting an explosive pull-up.

Exercise	Sets	Reps	Resistance (%)
Explosive Pull-ups	2	AMAP	BW
Wide Pull-ups	2	8	BW
Close Pull-ups	2	10	BW
Rest Periods		90 seconds between sets	

Workout 34
Sumo-Style

Class	Difficulty Level	Time
Power	Intermediate	30 minutes

There are only two exercises to complete in this workout; however, these two exercises complement each other well. While the sumo deadlift features the legs, lower back, and inner upper back muscles as prime movers, the wide grip pull-up requires the outer lats and biceps to function as the prime the movers while the legs and postural muscles function as stabilizers.

Exercise	Sets	Reps	Resistance (%)
Sumo Deadlift	5	5	75
Wide Pull-up	3	10	BW
Rest Periods		90 seconds between sets	

Workout 35
Power Back

Class	Difficulty Level	Time
Power	Advanced	30 minutes

It is incredibly important to use the proper form on this workout, as the back is more susceptible to injury than most other body parts. On the bent row, keep your chest up, head straight, and emphasize the natural arch in your back. Additionally, to perform a weighted pull-up simply place a weight belt around your waist and attached a chain connected to a 5, 10, or 25 pound weight plate to the end of it. If you are unable to complete weighted pull-ups, simply complete three sets of 6 bodyweight or assisted pull-ups.

Exercise	Sets	Reps	Resistance (%)
Deadlift	4	4	75
Pull-up (Weighted)	3	6	75
Bent Row	2	8	75
Rest Periods		90 seconds between sets	

Workout 36
Cleaning Up

Class	Difficulty Level	Time
Power	Advanced	30 minutes

This workout may seem like it would take longer than 30 minutes. However, because the first three exercises take place at the same workout station and because the rest periods are rather short, this workout can be done in roughly 30 minutes. Perform the bent row first while your lower back muscles are most fresh and take shorter rest periods between the shrug and pull-up sets. On the first exercise, the bent barbell row, perform the concentric portion of the lift as explosively as possible while keeping good form.

Exercise	Sets	Reps	Resistance (%)
Bent Row	4	4	75
Hang Clean	3	6	75
Power Shrug	3	8	75
Wide Pull-up	3	10	BW
Rest Periods		90 seconds between sets	

20

Back: Strength Workouts

Workout 37
Machine Strong

Class	Difficulty Level	Time
Strength	Beginner	20 minutes

This workout is meant to help you build strength in your back while using only machines and cables. This is a quick hitter, meaning that once you're in the gym, it should take no longer than 20 minutes. Although you will be going heavy, your rest periods will not be as long as they would be if you were doing free-weight exercises that forced you to stabilize. Safety is increased on this workout because you are only using machines and cables.

Exercise	Sets	Reps	Resistance (%)
Machine Row	2	6	75 - 85
Machine Pull-down	2	6	75 - 85
Seated Cable Row	2	8	75 - 80
Lat Pull-down	2	8	75 - 80
Rest Periods	60 - 90 seconds between sets		

Workout 38
Strong Pull

Class	Difficulty Level	Time
Strength	Beginner	30 minutes

This workout can be completed in even the sparsest of gyms. All you need is a pull-up bar and something to weigh you down on the first exercise. This will help you build strength primarily in your lats, the outer muscles of the back. However, the muscles of the middle and lower back and biceps will be targeted to some extent as well. Your abs, oblique and hip flexors will work to stabilize throughout the workout. Depending on your rest periods, this workout should not take longer than 25 minutes.

Exercise	Sets	Reps	Resistance
Wide Grip Pull-up	2	6	BW
Neutral Grip Pull-up	2	8	BW
Chin-up	2	8	BW
Rest Periods	60 - 90 seconds between sets		

Workout 39
Dumbbell Back Workout

Class	Difficulty Level	Time
Strength	Intermediate	30 minutes

This workout begins with a powerful unilateral dumbbell row. To perform this exercise grab a fairly heavy dumbbell and place it between your legs, which should be just wider than shoulder width apart with your right leg about six inches behind your left. Bend your torso over the weight and grab it with your right hand, with a neutral grip. With your back flat, chest up, and neck straight, explosively row the dumbbell up to your side, keeping your elbow in and hips even. After setting the weight back down, place it closer to the left leg, move the left leg back, and explosively row the weight with the left arm. That's one rep, complete four sets of 6 before moving onto a more traditional dumbbell row with both arms. Finish this workout with a bent over dumbbell raise.

Exercise	Sets	Reps	Resistance (%)
Dumbbell Row	4	6	85
Bent Dumbbell Raise	4	8	80
Rest Periods	60 - 90 seconds between sets		

Workout 40
Back Packed

Class	Difficulty Level	Time
Strength	Intermediate	30 minutes

This workout begins with a fairly heavy bent row, which is one of the most effective moves to develop strength not only in the back but throughout the entire body. In order to give the postural muscles of the lower back a break, wide grip pull-ups were added between the bent rows and the T-Bar rows.

Exercise	Sets	Reps	Resistance (%)
Bent Row	2	6	85
Wide Grip Pull-up	2	8	BW
T-Bar Row	2	8	80
Chin-up	2	8	BW
Rest Periods	60 - 90 seconds between sets		

22

Workout 41
Row Row Row

Class	Difficulty Level	Time
Strength	Advanced	30 minutes

This workout is primarily meant to challenge the muscles of the middle back, but it will certainly tax your lower and outer back muscles because they must stabilize throughout many of the exercises. Though the workout may seem redundant with this many rows, they all will hit the back muscles from different angles, meaning that while there will certainly be some overlap between the muscles fibers affected by the stimulus, various muscle fibers will be impacted during this workout.

Exercise	Sets	Reps	Resistance (%)
Bent Row	3	8	80
T-Bar Row	3	8	80
Standing Cable Row	2	8	80
Seated Cable Row	2	8	80
Rest Periods	60 - 90 seconds between sets		

Workout 42
Repeat Back

Class	Difficulty Level	Time
Strength	Advanced	30 minutes

This workout may look a bit familiar as it mirrors a similar workout; however, the reps are increased and the weight is decreased in this workout. Additionally, the rest period is slightly shortened here. This is done in order to transform the workout from one that focuses primarily on power to one that falls more into the spectrum of a "strength" workout. This shows that tinkering with sets, reps and rest periods can transform a workout from power to strength without changing the exercises.

Exercise	Sets	Reps	Resistance (%)
Bent Row	5	5	90
Hang Clean	4	8	85
Power Shrug	3	10	80
Wide Pull-up	2	12	BW
Rest Periods	60 - 90 seconds between sets		

Back: Muscle Building Workouts

Workout 43
Backed Up

Class	Difficulty Level	Time
Muscle Building	Beginner	25 minutes

To build back muscle you will use many of the same exercises and set protocols as prescribed in the power and strength building workouts. However, you will extend the rep ranges, use slightly lighter loads and shorten the rest periods. Because the rest periods are shorter and the weights are lighter, you will be able to fit more exercises and sets into a 30 minute window. Complete three sets of 8 -10 reps on each exercise.

Exercise	Sets	Reps	Resistance (%)
Bent Row	2	8	80
Wide Grip Pull-up	2	10	BW
Cable Row	2	10	75
Chin up	2	12	BW
Rest Periods		60- 90 seconds between sets	

Workout 44
Muscle Machine

Class	Difficulty Level	Time
Muscle Building	Beginner	30 minutes

In this workout, you are increasing sets and reps and reducing the weight load and rest periods of a previous workout in order to stimulate muscle growth rather than to work in a power or strength development range. This is an excellent way to still get in a great deal of volume when you do not have time to load free weights in the gym.

Exercise	Sets	Reps	Resistance (%)
Machine Row	3	8	80
Machine Pull-down	3	8	80
Seated Cable Row	3	10	75
Lat Pull-down	3	10	75
Rest Periods		60 seconds between sets	

Workout 45
All Around Awesome

Class	Difficulty Level	Time
Muscle Building	Intermediate	15 - 20 minutes

This back workout is meant to bring in as many different exercises and angels as possible in a 30 minute window. To complete the inverted row, simply lower a Smith Machine bar to 2 - 3 feet off of the ground and make sure that the safety hooks are securely fastened. Lay down flat on your back with the bar over your chest, and place your hands over the bar with an overhand grip. Pull your chest up to the bar with your legs and back flat and head straight. To add resistance to this exercise, have a spotter place a 10 or 25 pound weight plate on your chest before you begin your first set.

Exercise	Sets	Reps	Resistance (%)
Wide Grip Pull-up	3	10	BW
T-Bar Row	3	10	75
Close Grip Lat Pull-down	3	10	75
Inverted Pull-up	3	10	BW
Rest Periods		60 seconds between sets	

Workout 46
Big Foot Back

Class	Difficulty Level	Time
Muscle Building	Intermediate	30 minutes

This workout combines lighter sumo deadlifts with unilateral cable rows to hit the back from angles that you probably don't typically achieve in your normal routine. Use this workout to mix it up and spur on new muscle growth.

Exercise	Sets	Reps	Resistance (%)
Sumo	3	10	70
Single Arm T-Bar Row	3	10	75
Wide Grip Pull-up	2	10	75
Single Arm Lat Pull-down	2	10	75
Rest Periods		60 seconds between sets	

Workout 47
The 100 Pull-up Challenge

Class	Difficulty Level	Time
Muscle Building	Advanced	15 - 20 minutes

This is the 100 Pull-up challenge ... this means that you will complete 100 pull-ups in this workout. This is definitely one of the more advanced workouts in the back section, as you will need to have a solid background of pull-ups to be able to do it. The goal here is to complete ten sets of 10 pull-ups with 1 minute of rest between sets. Start with wide grip pull-ups, which are the most difficult, and then progress down to more and more narrow grips until you finally finish with chin-ups for the last two sets. A way to scale the workout down is to complete only one set per grip so that you complete 50 pull-ups in the workout.

Exercise	Sets	Reps	Resistance
Wide Pull-up	2	10	BW
Medium Pull-up	2	10	BW
Neutral Pull-up	2	10	BW
Close Pull-up	2	10	BW
Chin up	2	10	BW
Rest Periods		60 seconds between sets	

Workout 48
Pull the Pin

Class	Difficulty Level	Time
Muscle Building	Advanced	15 - 20 minutes

You will only complete two exercises in this workout; however, because of the lack of rest within the sets, this will still be very challenging. Start at the lat pull-down machine and pick a weight that allows you to complete 6, but no more than 6 reps. Complete the 6 reps then pull the pin, reset the weight to 20 pounds lighter, and complete 6 more reps. Rest one minute and repeat, and then do the same for the seated cable rows.

Exercise	Sets	Reps	Resistance (%)
Lat Pull-down	3	6 + 4	85 + 75
Cable Row	3	6 + 4	85 + 75
Rest Periods		60 seconds between sets	

Back: Endurance Workouts

Workout 49
Inverted Pull-up Burnout

Class	Difficulty Level	Time
Endurance	Intermediate	10 minutes

To set up this workout, adjust the smith machine bar to three feet off of the ground, make sure that the safety hooks are attached properly, and then lay down under the machine with the bar over your chest. Complete as many inverted rows as you can by touching your chest to the smith bar and then lowering yourself back down. When you fail, rest 10 – 15 seconds and complete as many as you can again. Do this for five sets total.

Exercise	Sets	Reps	Resistance
Inverted Pull-up	5	Varies	BW
Rest Periods		10 - 15 seconds between sets	

Workout 50
Pulled Up

Class	Difficulty Level	Time
Endurance	Beginner	30 minutes

The goal of this workout is to complete 20 pull-ups in the fewest number of sets as you can. Your overall goal should be to decrease the total number of sets that it takes to get to 20 from week to week until eventually you are able to complete 20 pull-ups in one set ... which would be pretty impressive.

Exercise	Sets	Reps	Resistance
Medium Pull-up	1 - 10	20	BW
Rest Periods		60 seconds between sets	

Workout 51
Super Back Set

Class	Difficulty Level	Time
Endurance	Intermediate	15 minutes

This workout is simply five rounds of 12 pull-ups followed immediately by 12 standing cable rows. To set this up, attach a hex handle to a cable pulley and lower the pulley to the lower quarter level. Perform 12 pull-ups, preferably wide-gripped, and then immediately pick up the pulley attachment and perform 12 standing rows. Remember to keep your head looking straight, chest up and back flat throughout the rows. It may help to use a stagger stance with one foot forward and one foot back in order to give you more stability while performing the rows.

Exercise	Sets	Reps	Resistance (%)
Wide Grip Pull-up	5	12	BW
Standing Cable Row	5	12	65
Rest Periods	60 seconds between sets		

Workout 52
Top to Bottom Row

Class	Difficulty Level	Time
Endurance	Intermediate	10 minutes

To complete this workout, place a hex handle or two D-handles to a cable apparatus and slide the cable attachment up to the top of the machine. Stand facing the cable apparatus with your feet slightly wider than shoulder width apart and grab the attachment with both hands. Row the cable towards your chest, hold for a second, and repeat. Complete 10 repetitions and then lower the pulley to the next rung down. Continue this sequence until the pulley is at the bottom rung of the apparatus. As you continue through the progression, continue to lower the weight as needed.

Exercise	Sets	Reps	Resistance (%)
Standing Cable Row	10	10	60
Rest Periods	10 seconds between sets		

Workout 53
The Pre-Exhaust

Class	Difficulty Level	Time
Endurance	Advanced	12 minutes

A pre-exhaust typically entails the use of a single joint exercise that targets a prime mover muscle but that does not target the stabilizer muscles typically associated with compound exercises that stimulate a particular muscle. For example, the prime movers in a chest press are the pectorals, and the main stabilizer muscles are the triceps and deltoids. A pre-exhaust for the pectorals would be a dumbbell fly because while it taxes those muscles, it does not target the triceps or deltoids. Here, you want to pre-exhaust the lats of the outer portion of the back without taxing the biceps, the forearms, and the abs. To do that, you will complete straight arm lat pull-downs immediately before pull-ups. You will notice that while completing the pull-ups, your arms feel more fresh than usual, but your back is fatiguing faster... this is what we are looking for.

Exercise	Sets	Reps	Resistance (%)
Straight Arm Lat-Pull-down	3	12	75
Wide Grip Pull-up	3	12	BW
Rest Periods	30 seconds between sets		

Workout 54
Lat Pull-down Pin Drop

Class	Difficulty Level	Time
Endurance	Advanced	12 minutes

This workout simply entails completing a running drop set of lat pull-downs. Choose a weight that you can complete 4, but only 4 reps and complete those reps. Pull the pin up to the next notch and complete 6 reps. Continue this sequence until you get to the very top weight and complete 2 more than the previous number of reps.

Exercise	Sets	Reps	Resistance (%)
Lat Pull-Down	2	4,6,8,10,12,14,16,18	Varies
Rest Periods	30 seconds between sets		

Back: Mixed Workouts

Workout 55
Mixed Back

Class	Difficulty Level	Time
Mixed	Beginner	30 minutes

This workout is primarily comprised of set and rep schemes that will promote hypertrophy and endurance; however, there will always be an overlap into power and strength to a certain extent. Follow the set and rep scheme for a well-rounded back workout.

Exercise	Sets	Reps	Resistance (%)
Plate Loaded Row	3	8 - 10	65 - 75
Wide Pull-down	3	10 - 12	60 - 70
Cable Row	3	12 - 15	50 - 65
Rest Periods		60 - 90 seconds between sets	

Workout 58
Lat Day

Class	Difficulty Level	Time
Mixed	Beginner	30 minutes

This workout is meant to target primarily the outer portion of your back. It is best to complete the pull-ups first and then the cable pull-downs because the pull-ups require far more stabilization than do lat pull-downs. As a general rule it is better to attack the exercises that require the most stabilization first in your workout and then move on to the exercises that do not require stabilization, such as pull-downs (with the exception of the pre-exhaust technique).

Exercise	Sets	Reps	Resistance (%)
Narrow Pull-up	2	8	BW
Lat Pull-down	2	12	60
Narrow Grip Lat Pull-down	2	12	60
Rest Periods		60 - 90 seconds between sets	

Workout 56
Back Stairs

Class	Difficulty Level	Time
Mixed	Intermediate	30 minutes

This workout contains one exercise each for power, strength, hypertrophy, and endurance. Use longer rest periods and heavier weight toward the beginning of the workout and shorter rest periods and lighter weight towards the end. You can use either a straight bar or a hex bar for the deadlifts. While either bar is sufficient for this exercise, the hex bar moves the center of mass of the weight back to the midline of your body, making it easier to keep your back flat throughout the lift.

Exercise	Sets	Reps	Resistance (%)
Deadlift	2	4	90
Wide Grip Pull-up	2	8	BW
Dumbbell Row	2	12	67
Lat Pull-down	2	15	65
Rest Periods		60 - 90 seconds between sets	

Workout 57
Row Day

Class	Difficulty Level	Time
Mixed	Intermediate	30 minutes

This workout is meant to emphasize the middle portion of your back focusing primarily on the trapezius and rhomboids. Like many of the other workouts in this section, it is best to use heavier weight and longer rest periods at the beginning of the workout and lighter weight with shorter rest periods towards the end.

Exercise	Sets	Reps	Resistance (%)
Bent Row	2	6	85
T-Bar Row	2	8	80
Plate Loaded Row	2	12	65
Cable Row	2	15	60
Rest Periods		60 - 90 seconds between sets	

Workout 59
Hanging Out

Class	Difficulty Level	Time
Mixed	Advanced	30 minutes

This workout starts out with a hang-clean. Although cleans are typically not necessarily thought of as back exercises, the hang clean is an excellent way to build power, strength, and size in the lower, middle and upper back. After the hang-cleans, complete two sets of wide grip pull-ups, followed by barbell shrugs and narrow grip lat pull-downs. The most difficult aspect of this workout may be maintaining grip strength throughout the first three exercises.

Exercise	Sets	Reps	Resistance (%)
Hang Clean	2	6	85
Wide Grip Pull-up	2	8	BW
Barbell Shrug	2	10	75
Narrow Lat Pull-down	2	12	67
Rest Periods	60 - 90 seconds between sets		

Workout 60
Back in Action

Class	Difficulty Level	Time
Mixed	Advanced	30 minutes

This is meant to be one of the most difficult back workouts in the book. This workout is heavy on explosive power exercises on the front end and moves more into hypertrophy and endurance building set and rep schemes on the back end. Take longer rest periods on the first two exercises, as they will require a great amount of energy and stabilization. The second two exercises lend themselves more to shorter rest periods and lighter weight.

Exercise	Sets	Reps	Resistance (%)
Clap Pull-ups	2	6	BW
Hang Clean	2	6	80
T-Bar Row	2	10	75
Lat Pull-downs	2	12	65
Rest Periods	60 - 90 seconds between sets		

32

Chapter 3

Shoulder Workouts

As with the back workouts, it is very difficult to isolate the shoulders in a workout, as most of the exercises will bring the muscles of the chest, back, core and triceps into play. Additionally, in order to prevent overuse injuries and to improve performance, it is important to program in such a way as to not work the same muscle groups back to back. For example, if you work out your chest on Monday, you may want to wait until Wednesday or Thursday to work out shoulders. This will give your front deltoids, triceps and upper chest time to recover before shoulder day. Additionally, because many people tend to work out their traps on shoulder day, many of the workouts in this section will feature workouts that target these muscles as well. Another key way to prevent injuries is to get a proper warm-up prior to beginning any of these workouts. In order to properly warm-up the shoulders, perform several cable or band resistance internal and external rotations, followed by a combination of overhead presses and raises. Many of the shoulder workouts do not have as much volume as some of the other muscle group workouts because of the need for increased warm-up time. Even still, these are excellent workouts to complete when you only have 30 minutes or less.

Workout 61
Power Dumbbell Shoulders

Class	Difficulty Level	Time
Power	Beginner	30 minutes

Begin this workout with a heavy seated overhead dumbbell press, followed by a heavy seated dumbbell shrug. Performing both of these exercises seated will keep you from cheating with your legs and will place more stress on the target muscle groups of the deltoids and the traps. Finish the workout with a standing cable upright row with a straight bar attachment to put further emphasis on your shoulders and traps.

Exercise	Sets	Reps	Resistance (%)
Seated Dumbbell Press	3	5	80
Seated Dumbbell Shrug	3	6	75
Cable Upright Row	3	8	70
Rest Periods	90 - 120 seconds between sets		

Workout 62
Super Shoulder Day

Class	Difficulty Level	Time
Power	Beginner	30 minutes

Although this is still a power workout featuring ten sets of military presses, adding the superman only helps to round off this workout and several others in this section if you have time to apply it. To perform the superman, grab a pair of light dumbbells that you could complete 25 lateral raises in one set with. From here, perform 10 lateral raises, followed immediately by 10 front raises, 10 external rotations with each arm, 10 cross raises and 10 bent over lateral raises.

Exercise	Sets	Reps	Resistance (%)
Military Press	10	5	50
Superman	1	60	Varies
Rest Periods	90 - 120 seconds between sets		

Workout 63
Boulder Shoulders

Class	Difficulty Level	Time
Power	Intermediate	30 minutes

This workout will help develop power throughout your entire body and is best completed with a spotter, as it begins with heavy military presses. You can use your legs to a small degree on the military press but incorporating them too much will equate to more of a jerk, which uses more momentum to carry the weight overhead. Here, you want to minimize momentum and keep most of the tension on the deltoids throughout the exercise. After the military presses, complete a barbell power shrug by loading the bar with 75% your 1RM and performing the reps as explosively as possible. Finish the workout with three sets of lateral dumbbell raises, which will further stress on your deltoids and traps.

Exercise	Sets	Reps	Resistance (%)
Military Press	5	5	70
Barbell Shrug	4	6	75
Lateral Raise	3	8	75
Rest Periods		90 - 120 seconds between sets	

Workout 64
All-Around Shoulder Power

Class	Difficulty Level	Time
Power	Intermediate	30 minutes

This workout begins with a barbell jerk; to perform this lift, un-rack the bar and hold it in front of you at the level of your front deltoids. Next, bend at the knees and hips slightly and then thrust the weight over your head in the form of a shoulder press using the momentum that you generated from your legs. After three sets of this, complete three sets of hang-cleans followed by standing dumbbell presses, one arm at a time.

Exercise	Sets	Reps	Resistance (%)
Barbell Split Jerk	3	5	75
Hang Clean	3	6	75
One arm Dumbbell Press	3	5 (Each Arm)	70
Rest Periods		90 - 120 seconds between sets	

Workout 65
Hang Clean Jerk

Class	Difficulty Level	Time
Power	Advanced	30 minutes

Complete five sets of 4 reps of hang clean and presses, followed by five sets of 5 reps of power shrugs. This workout is for advanced lifters who have a great deal of experience in the gym, and it should be done with a proper amount of rest between sets. This workout will place a great deal of stress on the lower back, core, and legs, so program your workouts accordingly. For instance, if you did a heavy back day that included deadlifts yesterday, don't try this workout today. This is a very explosive workout, as you are taking the bar straight from a hang clean into a jerk, which means that you will use your legs to explosively press the bar over your head once you have it in the top of the clean position. As for the power shrugs, place slightly more weight on the bar than you typically would for shrugs, and use your legs to explosively shrug the weight.

Exercise	Sets	Reps	Resistance (%)
Hang Clean and Press	5	4	75-85
Barbell Shrug	5	5	75-85
Rest Periods	90 - 120 seconds between sets		

Workout 66
Clean and Jerk Day

Class	Difficulty Level	Time
Power	Advanced	30 minutes

This workout is exactly as simple as it sounds. You will simply do ten sets of clean and jerks at 70% of your one rep max. The focus of this workout is speed and explosiveness. There is no need to go heavy here; just focus on performing each lift with perfect form and as much power as possible.

Exercise	Sets	Reps	Resistance (%)
Hang Clean and Jerk	10	5	70
Rest Periods	90 - 120 seconds between sets		

Shoulders: Strength Workouts

Workout 67
Dumbbell Strong

Class	Difficulty Level	Time
Strength	Beginner	25 minutes

This workout should have you in and out of the gym in a maximum of 25 minutes, as you will be able to jump immediately from exercise to exercise without traversing the entire gym. Begin by performing three sets of 6 dumbbell presses with each arm. Next, perform three sets of 8 dumbbell lateral raises, followed by three sets of 8 dumbbell shrugs.

Exercise	Sets	Reps	Resistance (%)
Dumbbell Press	3	6	85
Lateral Raise	3	8	80
Dumbbell Shrug	3	8	80
Rest Periods		90 - 120 seconds between sets	

Workout 68
Machine Shoulder Strength

Class	Difficulty Level	Time
Strength	Beginner	30 minutes

The machine shoulder strength workout allows you to load up the weight without worrying about stabilizing it as much, which gives you the opportunity to gain strength while minimizing the fear of injury. If your gym does not have a plate-loaded shoulder machine, begin with the smith machine press and then transition to a pin drop machine for the second exercise. Finish with a cable upright row followed by a cable shrug.

Exercise	Sets	Reps	Resistance (%)
Plate Loaded Shoulder Press	3	6	85
Smith Machine Shoulder Press	3	8	80
Cable Upright Row	2	8	80
Cable Shrug	2	8	80
Rest Periods		90 - 120 seconds between sets	

Workout 69
Fly Strong

Class	Difficulty Level	Time
Strength	Intermediate	30 minutes

Begin this workout with a cable front raise by attaching a straight bar attachment to the cable apparatus and facing away from the cable apparatus. Grasp the bar with an overhand grip and pull the cable through your legs. Raise the cable up so that your arms are parallel at 90 degrees at the top of the exercise. In order to perform the inverse cable fly, attach D-handles to both sides of a cable crossover machine and grab the left D-handle with your right hand and the right D-handle with your left hand. With arms crossed at the start, pull both sides across your body, finishing in an "X" pattern.

Exercise	Sets	Reps	Resistance (%)
Cable Front Raise	4	6	85
Lateral Raise	4	8	80
Inverted Cable Fly	3	8	80
Cable Shrug	2	8	80
Rest Periods		90 - 120 seconds between sets	

Workout 70
Smith Shoulder Strength

Class	Difficulty Level	Time
Strength	Intermediate	25 minutes

This workout will enable you to set up shop at the smith machine and stay there until your workout is done, which should only be around 25 minutes. A few things to be aware of for seated smith machine shoulder presses: first, be careful to set up an incline bench close enough to the smith machine bar to have a proper range of motion but far enough back so that you don't hit yourself in the chin or your nose when you press the bar up... that can be painful.

Exercise	Sets	Reps	Resistance (%)
Smith Press	4	8	80
Smith Shrug	4	8	80
Smith Upright Row	4	8	80
Rest Periods		90 - 120 seconds between sets	

Workout 71
All – Round Shoulder Strong

Class	Difficulty Level	Time
Strength	Advanced	25 minutes

This workout begins with the clean and jerk, which is a very taxing exercise in its own right, and ends with dumbbell raise exercises that each targets a different head of the deltoids. The front raise primarily targets the front deltoid, the lateral raise primarily targets the middle deltoid, and the bent over raise primarily targets the rear deltoid. Although these raises target the individual muscles that form the majority of the shoulder, each of these exercises will have an impact on all of the muscles in the shoulder and on the trapezius as well.

Exercise	Sets	Reps	Resistance (%)
Clean and Jerk	4	6	80
Front Raise	2	8	80
Lateral Raise	2	8	80
Bent Raise	2	8	80
Rest Periods	90 - 120 seconds between sets		

Workout 72
Military Press Muscle

Class	Difficulty Level	Time
Strength	Intermediate	20 minutes

This is an excellent workout for building upper body strength when you are limited on time because you won't leave the rack. Remember that military presses are meant to be performed more strictly than push-presses or jerks, which place most of the resistance on the deltoids and triceps. Progress slowly with this exercise; only add weight once you can successfully finish the entire 6 rep protocol with your current weight.

Exercise	Sets	Reps	Resistance (%)
Military Press	5	6	80
Barbell Shrug	4	8	80
Rest Periods	90 - 120 seconds between sets		

Shoulders: Muscle Building Workouts

Workout 73
Shoulder Machine Growth

Class	Difficulty Level	Time
Muscle Building	Beginner	20 minutes

This workout is comprised of three quick-hitting machine moves that are excellent for gaining size without the need of a spotter. This workout should only take around 20 minutes, as the rest periods will be shorter than would be necessary for free weight exercises.

Exercise	Sets	Reps	Resistance (%)
Plate Loaded Shoulder Press	2	10	75
Standing Smith Machine Press	2	10	75
Shoulder Machine Press	2	10	75
Rest Periods	60 seconds between sets		

Workout 74
Dumbbell Shoulder Size

Class	Difficulty Level	Time
Muscle Building	Beginner	20 minutes

Because you will only be working at the dumbbell rack, this workout does not require much time spent in between sets loading up bars or scouring the entire gym for a free machine. Begin this workout with either standing or seated dumbbell military presses and finish it with either standing or seated dumbbell shrugs.

Exercise	Sets	Reps	Resistance (%)
Dumbbell Shoulder Press	2	10	65 - 75
Lateral Raise	2	10	65 - 75
Front Raise	2	10	65 - 75
Bent Raise	2	10	65 - 75
Dumbbell Shrug	2	10	65 - 75
Rest Periods	60 - 90 seconds between sets		

Workout 75
All-Around Shoulder Blaster

Class	Difficulty Level	Time
Muscle Building	Intermediate	25 minutes

Begin this workout with a standing military press, completing three sets of 10 reps followed by the next three exercises as a compound set, which means that you will perform the exercises back to back to back with only as much rest as is necessary to move the weight into position for the next exercise. On the EZ Bar exercises, use your 10 rep max weight for the front raise, as it is the most difficult exercise in this progression.

Exercise	Sets	Reps	Resistance (%)
Military Press	3	10	75
EZ Bar Upright Row	2	10	75
EZ Bar Front Raise	2	10	70
EZ Arnold Press	2	10	70
Dumbbell Shrug	2	10	65
Rest Periods	60 seconds between sets		

Workout 76
Shoulder Cable Growth

Class	Difficulty Level	Time
Muscle Building	Intermediate	30 minutes

Begin this workout by attaching a straight bar attachment to a cable crossover machine and performing standing military presses with that attachment. Next, using the same attachment but less resistance, perform a standing upright row with the cable machine. After this, perform a between the legs cable front raise followed by a cable face pull in order to target the rear deltoid muscles as well as the muscles in the middle of your back.

Exercise	Sets	Reps	Resistance (%)
Cable Press	3	10	75
Cable Upright Row	2	10	75
Cable Front Raise	2	10	75
Cable Face Pull	2	10	75
Cable Shrug	2	10	75
Rest Periods	60 seconds between sets		

Workout 77
Military Press Pyramid

Class	Difficulty Level	Time
Muscle Building	Advanced	30 minutes

The military pyramid workout will help you gain strength and size in your shoulders by taking you through various rep and weight ranges within the first exercise. After a thorough warm-up, begin by loading a straight bar with 75% of your 1RM for military press and completing ten reps with strict form. Work your way up in weight and down in reps on the next set, where you will be using 80% of your 1RM to complete 8 reps. You will reach the peak of the pyramid on the third set, where you will complete six reps of 85% of your 1RM. After this, you will progress back down in weight and back up in reps until you reach the weight and rep range that you began with on your fifth set.

Exercise	Sets	Reps	Resistance (%)
Military Press	5	10,8,6,8,10	75,80,85,80,75
Lateral Raise	2	10	75
Barbell Shrug	2	10	75
Rest Periods		60 - 90 seconds between sets	

Workout 78
Military Pressed

Class	Difficulty Level	Time
Muscle Building	Advanced	20 minutes

Simply complete ten sets of 10 reps of the military press. Here, choose a weight that you could complete one set of 25 - 30 reps with. Try to use this weight throughout the workout, but if your form begins to break down and you have to use momentum to finish your lifts, lower the weight and continue. This workout is meant to be completed only rarely because it could lead to overtraining. As long as you maintain proper form and warm up and cool down appropriately, this workout is an excellent choice to shock your muscles into new growth.

Exercise	Sets	Reps	Resistance (%)
Military Press	10	10	60
Rest Periods		60 seconds between sets	

Shoulders: Endurance Workouts

Workout 79
Shoulder Pin Drop

Class	Difficulty Level	Time
Endurance	Beginner	15 minutes

Shoulder Pin Drop is a shoulder press workout that can be used as a series of intervals or as a burnout within a larger workout. Begin with a weight that only allows you to complete 4 reps. Once you finish 4 reps, immediately pull the pin and place it on the next lightest weight and perform 6 reps. Continue this trend, pulling up the pin and placing it on the next lightest setting while completing 2 additional reps with each pull until you have completed ten total sets. If you are using this as a burnout, you will be finished after the tenth set, but if you are using this as your entire workout, rest for four minutes and then start the entire sequence over at 4, this time using the weight that you used for either the second or third set for your first set.

Exercise	Sets	Reps	Resistance(%)
Shoulder Press Machine	10	4,6,8,10,12,14,16,18,20,22	Varies
Rest Periods	90 seconds between sets		

Workout 80
Shoulder Marathon

Class	Difficulty Level	Time
Endurance	Beginner	20 minutes

This workout, like many others in the endurance section, is meant to be completed as a circuit with little to no rest between the various exercises. Complete a single set of each exercise, rest 90 seconds, and then complete each exercise again.

Exercise	Sets	Reps	Resistance (%)
Lateral Raise	2	10	50
Front Raise	2	10	50
Bent Raise	2	10	50
Overhead Raise	2	10	50
Rest Periods	90 seconds between sets		

Workout 81
The Wheel

Class	Difficulty Level	Time
Endurance	Intermediate	5 minutes

To set this workout up, grab a 45 pound plate, a 35 pound plate, a 25 pound plate, and a 10 pound plate and place them next to each other on a flat bench. Stand next to the bench and grasp the 45 pound plate with your hands directly across from each other on each side of the plate. First, perform a wheel turn by raising the plate directly in front of your face and then twisting the plate like a steering wheel side to side. When both hands have been on "top" of the weight, you have completed one rep. Once you have completed 10 reps, move on to a front raise with the same weight plate.

Exercise	Sets	Reps	Resistance (lbs.)
Plate Wheel/Raise	1	10	45
Plate Wheel/Raise	1	10	35
Plate Wheel/Raise	1	10	25
Plate Raise/Wheel	1	10	10
Rest Periods	5 seconds between sets		

Workout 82
Running the Fixed Rack

Class	Difficulty Level	Time
Endurance	Intermediate	12 - 15 minutes

The typical rack of fixed barbells features barbells that weigh 10 – 100 pounds, increasing in 10 pound increments. To start, grab the 100 pound barbell (or the heaviest you can handle for 4 reps with good form) and complete 4 reps of standing shoulder press. Immediately rack the weight and grab the 90 pound barbell and complete 6 reps. Continue all the way to the lightest barbell on the rack and rep out the requisite number of reps. If you decide that you can complete two rounds of this, slash the number of reps in half on the second round so that you begin with 2 reps rather than 4.

Exercise	Sets	Reps	Resistance (%)
Fixed Barbell Shoulder Press	2	4,6,8,10,12,14,16,18, 20	Varies
Rest Periods	90 seconds between sets		

Workout 83
Fives

Class	Difficulty Level	Time
Endurance	Advanced	15 minutes

The Five's workout is a shoulder circuit that will help you develop power and endurance in your shoulders and throughout your upper body. Begin by choosing a weight that you would consider to be 50% of your 1RM for the hang clean and press. Next, perform 5 upright rows, followed immediately by 5 hang-cleans, 5 push presses and 5 shrugs. Use an overhand grip, placing your hands about shoulder width apart on the bar, and do not rest in between the different exercises. This is an excellent way to increase power for a longer period of contraction.

Exercise	Sets	Reps	Resistance (%)
Barbell Upright Row	3	5	50
Hang Clean	3	5	50
Barbell Push Press	3	5	50
Barbell Shrug	3	5	50
Rest Periods	90 seconds between sets		

Workout 84
Smith Swap

Class	Difficulty Level	Time
Endurance	Advanced	12 - 15 minutes

To begin, load the bar with a 45 lb. plate (or 35 or 25) on each side. Stand facing the smith machine and un-rack the weight from the safeties in a shoulder press position. Perform 8 shoulder presses, then rack the weight and immediately replace the 45 lb. plates with 35 lb. plates and perform 10 more smith presses. Once you finish those, immediately replace the 35 lb. plates with 25's to perform a set of 12 reps, and subsequently use 10 lb. plates to complete a set of 15 reps. You may need to start lighter than the 45's, depending on your strength level.

Exercise	Sets	Reps	Resistance (Lbs.)
Standing Smith Shoulder Press	3	8,10,12,15	45, 35, 25, 10
Rest Periods	90 seconds between sets		

Shoulders: Mixed Workouts

Workout 85
Shoulder Smith

Class	Difficulty Level	Time
Mixed	Beginner	25 minutes

If you have a very limited amount of time but still want to get in a great shoulder workout, try the Shoulder Smith workout. Here, all you need is a smith machine and you're in business. Begin by performing standing smith machine overhead shoulder presses. Next, transition into an upright row; this will require that you significantly reduce the amount of weight that you are using. Finally, perform shrugs on the smith machine to push the endurance of your traps. Once again, this workout requires longer rest periods at the beginning and shorter rest periods as the workout progresses.

Exercise	Sets	Reps	Resistance (%)
Smith Shoulder Press	3	8	60
Smith Upright Row	3	12	70
Smith Shrug	3	15	50
Rest Periods	60 - 90 seconds between sets		

Workout 86
Mixed Machine Shoulders

Class	Difficulty Level	Time
Mixed	Beginner	25 minutes

Begin this machine-only workout with a heavy plate-loaded shoulder press with long rest periods. Next, move on to the smith machine and perform three sets of shrugs with moderate weight, reps, and rest periods. Finish by performing isolated shoulder raises with light weight and short rest periods.

Exercise	Sets	Reps	Resistance (%)
Plate Loaded Shoulder Press	3	6	60
Smith Shrug	3	8	70
Shoulder Raise	3	12	50
Rest Periods	60-90 seconds between sets		

Workout 87
Bar Shoulders

Class	Difficulty Level	Time
Mixed	Intermediate	30 minutes

If you are looking for a shoulder workout that will help develop your power, strength, endurance, and add muscle mass, all within 30 minutes, this is it. It may seem as though this workout has too much volume for it to be completed in 30 minutes but because all of the exercises will take place in the same place, with the same bar, it is feasible to finish workout in 25 minutes or so. Rest longer (90 – 120 seconds) between sets on the hang clean and presses and then shorten the rest periods on the subsequent exercises.

Exercise	Sets	Reps	Resistance (%)
Hang Clean and Press	3	5	70
Barbell Shrug	3	8	80
Upright Row	3	10	60
Barbell Front Raise	3	15	50
Rest Periods	60 - 90 seconds between sets		

Workout 88
Delt Driver

Class	Difficulty Level	Time
Mixed	Intermediate	30 minutes

This workout strengthens all three of your shoulder heads by incorporating a mix of dumbbell and EZ bar moves. The intermittent upright rows, both with dumbbells and an EZ bar, serve as a pre-exhaust for the presses that follow. This is an excellent way to push your shoulders to fatigue.

Exercise	Sets	Reps	Resistance (%)
Dumbbell Shoulder Press	3	8	70
Upright Row	2	15	80
EZ Arnold Press	3	10	60
EZ Upright Row	2	15	40
Fixed Barbell Press	3	10	40
Rest Periods	60 - 90 seconds between sets		

Workout 89
Clean and Jerk Day

Class	Difficulty Level	Time
Mixed	Advanced	30 minutes

Begin by placing 60% of your 1RM on a straight bar. Perform two sets of 5 clean and jerks with 90 seconds of rest between sets. Next, grab a pair of dumbbells and perform two sets of the same exercise. Dumbbell clean and jerks may be difficult to get used to because, unlike a straight bar, the handles do not swivel. If this is the first time you are going to attempt them be sure to go light, using a weight that allows you to maintain proper form. Last, complete an alternating unilateral kettle bell clean and press.

Exercise	Sets	Reps	Resistance (%)
Clean and Jerk	2	5	60
Dumbbell Clean and Jerk	2	8	60
Kettlebell Clean and Press	2	16 (8 each side)	60
Rest Periods	60-90 seconds between sets		

Workout 90
Shoulder Knockout

Class	Difficulty Level	Time
Mixed	Advanced	30 minutes

This workout is meant to help develop a range of strength, hypertrophy, and endurance in your shoulders. Begin with the military press, as it is a heavy free weight exercise and requires the largest amount of stabilization. To increase the intensity, complete these moves in superset fashion, performing a set of raises immediately following each set of presses.

Exercise	Sets	Reps	Resistance (%)
Military Press	2	6	80
Front Raise	2	12	60
Plate Loaded Shoulder Press	2	8	70
Lateral Raise	2	12	60
Smith Shoulder Press	2	10	60
Bent Raise	2	12	60
Rest Periods	60 - 90 seconds between sets		

Chapter 4

Lower Body Workouts

Regardless of your goals, working the lower body is a critical aspect of any training program, as the muscles in the legs are the largest in the body. Because of the relatively large cross-sectional area of the muscle in the legs, training them can elicit a stronger acute release of muscle building hormones, which can aid significantly to gains in muscular strength and size (10). Once you begin training your legs, you will notice that your power, strength, size, and endurance will increase throughout the entire body, not just your lower body. I know that leg day is by far the easiest day to skip, but if you really want to see major improvement, you will find a way to stay motivated to get to the squat rack. A key thought to keep in mind is that with any type of training, be it lower or upper body, consistency is the key. As for the various sections in this chapter, remember that training for power, particularly lower body and whole body power, typically requires expertise, or at least competency in rather complicated and challenging exercises such as squats, deadlifts, and power cleans. Because these moves are difficult to master and require the instruction of an experienced personal trainer or strength coach, beginner workouts will feature mostly body-weight and machine exercises, even though they may not always be the most efficient for lower body power, strength, and hypertrophy development. If you are a beginner and want to perform exercises such as the weighted back squat or , I recommend finding an experienced, credentialed trainer to work with you on your form. Once you feel comfortable and confident in performing these moves correctly, you can start to incorporate more complex lifts into your workouts. For now, however, the "Beginner" sections will feature exercises that are relatively safer for a newbie to try. Like the other chapters, the expected finish time of these workouts is an estimate and does not include warmup time. It is very important to warmup on leg day, as many of the exercises are compound in nature and bring into play many different muscles groups. A good warmup on leg day could include a short round of cardio along with bodyweight and light squats, lunges, and deadlifts.

Lower Body: Power Workouts

Workout 91
Jump Day

Class	Difficulty Level	Time
Power	Beginner	30 minutes

Set this workout up by finding a plyometric (plyo) box that you feel confident that you can jump onto with two feet. Complete four sets of 4 reps with 90 seconds of rest between reps. Next, using only your bodyweight, perform three sets of 6 jump squats. While performing the squat portion of the jump squat, focus on keeping your weight on your heels both on the way down and back up. Once you reach the top portion of the movement, transfer your weight to your toes and jump up as explosively as possible. Finish the workout with standing calf raises.

Exercise	Sets	Reps	Resistance
Box Jump	4	4	BW
Jump Squat	3	6	BW
Standing Calf Raise	2	8	BW
Rest Periods		2 minutes between sets	

Workout 92
Squat Power

Class	Difficulty Level	Time
Power	Beginner	30 minutes

Here, complete two variations of the squat followed by a plyometric box jump. Be sure to take adequate rest periods, particularly on the box jumps, as these are meant to be a power rather than endurance exercise in this workout. You don't need to go very heavy here; just focus on performing each rep explosively but with perfect form.

Exercise	Sets	Reps	Resistance (%)
Back Squat	2	4	70
Front Squat	2	4	70
Plyo Box Jump	2	4	BW
Rest Periods		2 minutes between sets	

Workout 93
Power Leg Day

Class	Difficulty Level	Time
Power	Intermediate	30 minutes

Begin this workout with a jump squat with very light weight. Fixed barbells lend themselves very well to this exercise, as they are more stable than a typical barbell that you would load. Next, perform light sumo deadlifts, where you will place your feet even with the outside rings on a loaded barbell and grasp the barbell with a narrow alternated grip. Raise the barbell in a smooth motion, keeping your back flat, chest up, and head straight. Finish the workout with three sets of 4 plyometric box jumps. There is a great deal of confusion around the use of the box jump these days as a result of the move being performed as a cardiovascular exercise rather than as a plyometric exercise in various workout programs. These workouts would prescribe sets of multiple repeated reps with little rest between sets.

Exercise	Sets	Reps	Resistance (%)
Jump Squat	4	5	30
Sumo	2	8	60
Plyo Box Jump	3	4	BW
Rest Periods		2 minutes between sets	

Workout 94
Explosion

Class	Difficulty Level	Time
Power	Intermediate	30 minutes

Begin this explosive workout with five sets of power cleans for 4 reps. Next, progress to a plyometric box jump and finish with a body weight squat jump. Use long rest periods between sets and focus on form throughout each lift, as these moves expose you to greater risk if done incorrectly.

Exercise	Sets	Reps	Resistance (%)
Power Clean	4	4	75-85
Plyo Box Jump	3	4	75-85
Squat Jump	2	6	BW
Rest Periods		2 minutes between sets	

orkout 95
Functional Power

Class	Difficulty Level	Time
Power	Advanced	30 minutes

This workout entails the use of only a barbell, plates, and a squat rack, which is all you need to develop total body power. Begin this workout with heavy back squats and then move to heavy deadlifts. Feel free to use a hex bar on the deadlifts if your gym has one; otherwise simply un-rack the bar you used for squats. Finish the workout with two sets of front squats followed by two sets of sumo deadlifts.

Exercise	Sets	Reps	Resistance (%)
Squat	4	4	75-85
Deadlift	4	4	75-85
Front Squat	2	6	75-85
Sumo	2	6	75-85
Rest Periods		2 minutes between sets	

Workout 96
Dead Power

Class	Difficulty Level	Time
Power	Advanced	30 minutes

This workout begins with a standard deadlift and is followed immediately by a sumo deadlift and a cable pull-through. To perform a cable pull-through, attach a rope attachment to the pulley and lower the pulley to the very bottom of the cable machine. Stand with your back to the cable machine and bend over into a bent row position, with your back flat, chest up, head straight, and feet just wider than shoulder width. Grasp the ropes with an inverted grip, with the knuckles of each hand facing each other. Extend at the hips and raise your chest up to a standing position, all the while gripping the rope but not extending your arms. Once you have slowly lowered the cable under control, you have completed one rep.

Exercise	Sets	Reps	Resistance (%)
Deadlift	4	4	75-85
Sumo	3	6	75-85
Cable Pull Through	2	8	75-85
Rest Periods		2 minutes between sets	

Lower Body: Strength Workouts

Workout 97
Strong Legs

Class	Difficulty Level	Time
Strength	Beginner	30 minutes

This is an excellent workout for the development of overall lower body strength. This workout begins with squats because squats require the greatest amount of muscles and should be completed before single joint exercises. Next, incorporate leg extensions and leg curls as either single sets or super sets. If you are looking to add intensity and/or to save time, perform the extensions and curls as a superset with little to no rest between each set.

Exercise	Sets	Reps	Resistance (%)
Squat	4	6	75 - 85
Leg Extension	2	8	80
Leg Curl	2	8	80
Rest Periods			90 seconds between sets

Workout 98
Machine Magic

Class	Difficulty Level	Time
Strength	Beginner	30 minutes

Machine Magic allows you to work on strengthening your legs without bringing stability into the equation. The only squat variation in this workout is the smith front squat, which does not require a spotter, making this a good workout if you are heading to the gym by yourself. While you certainly do need to learn and master free weight exercises, this workout is a relatively safe bet to help you gain strength while you are still perfecting free-weight lifts.

Exercise	Sets	Reps	Resistance (%)
Machine Leg Press	3	5	85
Smith Front Squat	3	5	80
Leg Extension	2	6	80
Leg Curl	2	6	80
Rest Periods			90 seconds between sets

Workout 99
Leg 5's

Class	Difficulty Level	Time
Strength	Intermediate	30 minutes

This workout is as simple as it looks. Perform five sets of 5 reps on both squats and deadlifts. It is critical that you keep your back flat, chest up, and head looking straight throughout each of these lifts, as these are two of the most taxing exercises you can perform. While this workout does not contain a ton of volume, it is still very taxing on the entire body because of the nature of these lifts and the loads that you will use.

Exercise	Sets	Reps	Resistance (%)
Squat	5	5	85
Deadlift	5	5	85
Rest Periods		90 seconds between sets	

Workout 100
100th Workout

Class	Difficulty Level	Time
Strength	Intermediate	30 minutes

Begin the 100th workout with a heavy squat for three straight sets, followed by a heavy deadlift. Next, progress to weighted step-ups followed by weighted lunges and calf raises. Here, once again, you can increase the intensity and turn this more into a hypertrophy/endurance workout by super-setting the step-ups and lunges, which will also decrease the time required to complete this workout. Notice also that this is the first leg workout that features calf raises. That is not because the calves are not important; every part of the body is important. The reason is that within a 30 minute time frame sometimes direct calf work simply becomes the odd exercise out.

Exercise	Sets	Reps	Resistance (%)
Squat	3	5	85
Deadlift	3	5	85
Step-up	2	6	80
Lunge	2	6	80
Calf Raise	2	8 (Each Leg)	75
Rest Periods		90 seconds between sets	

54

Workout 101
Dead Strength

Class	Difficulty Level	Time
Strength	Advanced	30 minutes

This workout places an emphasis on the hamstrings on the "back" side of the leg. It is important to work both sides of the leg to develop strength evenly in order to improve performance and prevent injury. However, it is OK to occasionally focus primarily on one side of the leg, particularly if you plan to spend another day working the other side. Try this workout during a week in which you can complete a front-dominant workout later in the week.

Exercise	Sets	Reps	Resistance (%)
Deadlift	4	6	85
Sumo Deadlift	3	8	80
Cable Pull Through	2	10	75
Rest Periods		90 seconds between sets	

Workout 102
Squat Strength

Class	Difficulty Level	Time
Strength	Advanced	30 minutes

This workout begins with the back squat and progresses through the front squat and box jump. Throughout the workout, focus on keeping the majority of your weight on your heels rather than on your toes, with the exception of the top of the extension phase of the box jumps. The rest periods may be slightly shorter than what you are used to for a box jump, but 90 seconds should be sufficient rest.

Exercise	Sets	Reps	Resistance (%)
Back Squat	4	6	75-85
Front Squat	4	8	75-85
Box Jump	4	6	BW
Rest Periods		90 seconds between sets	

Lower Body: Muscle Building Workouts

Workout 104
Back Side Boost

Class	Difficulty Level	Time
Muscle Building	Beginner	30 minutes

If you're looking to build your backside, this is your workout. Perform stiff-legged deadlifts as your second exercise, keeping your knees close to locked out but not entirely so. Be especially careful here to keep your head straight, chest up, and back flat. After completing two sets of step-ups, drop the weight and complete two sets of walking lunges using only your bodyweight.

Exercise	Sets	Reps	Resistance (%)
Squat	2	10	75
Stiff-Legged	2	10	75
Step Up	2	10	BW
Walking Lunge	2	40 Yards	BW
Rest Periods		90 seconds between sets	

Workout 105
Machine Legs

Class	Difficulty Level	Time
Muscle Building	Beginner	30 minutes

Begin this workout with a fairly heavy smith machine front squat, then progress to leg presses, leg extensions, and finish with leg curls. Because you are beginning with front squats, your quads will be more fatigued than your glutes and hamstrings on the leg press. To account for this, place your feet a bit higher on the leg press platform; this will place more emphasis on the muscles of the back side of the body, which are often neglected.

Exercise	Sets	Reps	Resistance (%)
Smith Front Squat	4	10	75
Leg Press	4	10	75
Leg Extension	2	10	75
Leg Curl	2	10	75
Rest Periods		90 seconds between sets	

Workout 106
Superset Front Squat/Lunge

Class	Difficulty Level	Time
Muscle Building	Intermediate	30 minutes

To perform this workout, grab a fixed barbell that is only moderately heavy. Perform 10 front squats, keeping your head and neck straight, elbows at 90 degrees, back flat, and chest up. Next, immediately press the weight overhead and onto your back. Perform 10 stationary lunges with each leg. That's one set. Perform five sets. Be sure to clear the space around you in the gym, as you do not want to lose balance and run into any stray weights on the gym floor.

Exercise	Sets	Reps	Resistance (%)
Front Squat	5	10	50
Lunges	5	10	50
Rest Periods	90 seconds between sets		

Workout 107
Squat Size

Class	Difficulty Level	Time
Muscle Building	Intermediate	30 minutes

This simple workout is highly effective in a time crunch, as it allows you to work a large amount of muscle groups in only eight sets. The back squats will allow you to use heavier weight than the front squats so complete them first when you are fresh. Be sure to keep your elbows pointing straight ahead on the front squats while your back is flat and chest is out. Although it is difficult not to lean forward on this exercise, try to keep most of the weight on your heels as you complete your reps.

Exercise	Sets	Reps	Resistance (%)
Back Squat	4	10	75
Front Squat	4	10	75
Rest Periods	90 seconds between sets		

Workout 108
Machine Mass

Class	Difficulty Level	Time
Muscle Building	Advanced	30 minutes

This workout can get you out of a pinch if you're looking to add mass to the wheels but are missing a spotter. Begin with the smith machine squat followed by the plate-loaded leg press. Next, perform the leg curls and leg extensions as a superset, resting only as long as necessary to change out the equipment or to move from one machine to the next.

Exercise	Sets	Reps	Resistance (%)
Smith Machine Squat	3	10	75
Plate Loaded Leg Press	3	10	75
Leg Curl	3	10	75
Leg Extension	3	10	75
Rest Periods		90 seconds between sets	

Workout 109
Squat All Day

Class	Difficulty Level	Time
Muscle Building	Advanced	30 minutes

Here, begin with a weight that is very easy, around 10% of your 1RM that you would normally use for a warm-up. Perform a set of 10 reps with this light weight and then add 10 pounds to the bar. Continue until you get to the sixth set, where you will keep the same amount of weight on the bar as was used on the fifth. Perform 10 reps of this weight for the sixth set, and then take 10 pounds off for the seventh set. Continue taking 10 pounds off until you finish set ten. Getting the weight right at the beginning is the tricky part, but after some trial and error, you should be ready to go!

Exercise	Sets	Reps	Resistance (%)
Back Squat	10	10	Varies
Rest Periods		90 seconds between sets	

Lower Body: Muscular Endurance Workouts

Workout 110
Walking Lunge

Class	Difficulty Level	Time
Endurance	Beginner	30 minutes

This workout can be used as the capstone exercise following a strength or hypertrophy workout or it can be used as a quick endurance workout. If you don't have time to get to the gym, you could even do this in an office hallway to get a quick leg workout in. Try this with only your body weight first and then progress to light weight once you are able to complete it with ease without weight.

Exercise	Sets	Reps	Resistance (%)
Walking Lunge	5	20	BW
Rest Periods	2 minutes between sets		

Workout 111
Step-up Day

Class	Difficulty Level	Time
Endurance	Beginner	30 minutes

If you're really into hiking but the weather is preventing you from getting outdoors, this workout may be for you. Train yourself to be ready to climb mountains by grabbing a 12 or 18 inch plyo box and placing it in an open area of the gym. Step up onto to the box with your lead leg and then bring up the rear leg to meet it atop the platform. Step back down with the original rear leg followed by the original lead leg. That's one rep. Next, replicate the previous sequence but reverse the roles of each leg, meaning that the original lead leg is now the rear leg and vice versa. Complete five sets of 20 reps with each leg with no weight. Once you are able to easily complete this, grab a light set of dumbbells or a weighted vest or backpack and complete the workout.

Exercise	Sets	Reps	Resistance (%)
Bodyweight Step Up	5	20	BW
Rest Periods	2 minutes between sets		

Workout 112
Lunge/Step-up Burnout

Class	Difficulty Level	Time
Endurance	Intermediate	30 minutes

This workout can either be performed as a burnout at the end of a strength or muscle building workout, or it can be used as a quick muscular endurance workout on its own. Here, simply use your bodyweight to complete lunges followed immediately by step-ups. Complete four sets of 20 reps of this superset with no rest between the two exercises.

Exercise	Sets	Reps	Resistance (%)
Bodyweight Lunge	4	20	75
Bodyweight Step Up	4	20	75
Rest Periods	90 seconds between sets		

Workout 113
Calf Superset

Class	Difficulty Level	Time
Endurance	Advanced	30 minutes

Begin this workout by loading a fairly heavy amount of weight onto the seated calf machine and complete a set of 15 reps. Immediately jump up and find a standing calf raise machine; complete 15 reps of standing calf raise and then rest. Repeat this sequence four more times for an excellent calf burnout that hits both muscles that comprise the calf, the soleus and the gastrocnemius.

Exercise	Sets	Reps	Resistance (%)
Seated Calf Raise	5	15	60
Standing Calf Raise	5	15	60
Rest Periods	2 minutes between sets		

Workout 114
Leg Extension / Leg Curl

Class	Difficulty Level	Time
Endurance	Advanced	30 minutes

I am a big believer in using exercises like squats and deadlifts when training the lower body because these moves incorporate larger muscle groups and require stabilization, which means they help you build more strength and burn more calories than their isolation exercise counterparts. However, there is certainly a time and place to incorporate these isolation moves into a workout, particularly toward the end of a workout that includes more compound moves. Here, the idea is to superset leg extensions and leg curls, using light weight and resting minimally between sets. This exercise sequence can be used as a finisher to a longer workout or as its own complete workout.

Exercise	Sets	Reps	Resistance (%)
Leg Extension	5	15	55
Leg Curl	5	15	55
Rest Periods	2 minutes between sets		

Workout 115
Body Weight Squat Challenge

Class	Difficulty Level	Time
Endurance	Advanced	30 minutes

The body weight squat challenge is similar to both the push-up challenge and the pull-up challenge. Perform this workout when you are on the road and don't have a gym at your disposal. The goal is to perform 100 body weight squats in as few sets as possible in as little time as possible. If you are able to perform 100 body weight squats in a row, progress to 125, 150, and then 200.

Exercise	Sets	Reps	Resistance (%)
Body Weight Squat	As few as possible	100	BW
Rest Periods	20 seconds between sets		

Lower Body: Mixed Workouts

Workout 116
Leg Day

Class	Difficulty Level	Time
Mixed	Beginner	30 minutes

This is an excellent lower body workout that features a variety of both functional and machine based exercises. Use longer rest periods and heavier loads at the beginning of the workout while you perform squats and lunges and then progress to shorter rest periods and lighter weight as you move down to leg extensions and leg curls.

Exercise	Sets	Reps	Resistance (%)
Squat	2	6	70 - 80
Deadlift	2	6	70 - 80
Bodyweight Lunges	2	8	BW
Leg Extension	2	10 - 12	55
Leg Curl	2	10 - 12	55
Rest Periods	Varies		

Workout 117
Function Day

Class	Difficulty Level	Time
Mixed	Beginner	30 minutes

Workouts such as this will help you develop strength, size, and endurance throughout your lower body, which can in turn build more muscle and burn more body fat than single joint moves (2). This workout will be particularly taxing on your lower back, so be sure to perform this workout when you are fresh and focus on using good form throughout the workout.

Exercise	Sets	Reps	Resistance (%)
Squat	2	6 - 8	70
Deadlift	2	6 - 8	70
Front Squat	2	10 - 12	50
Sumo	2	10 - 12	50
Rest Periods	2 minutes		

Workout 118
Day of the Dead... Lift

Class	Difficulty Level	Time
Mixed	Intermediate	20 minutes

This is an example of how you can use a single exercise to achieve gains in power, strength, hypertrophy, and endurance in a workout. Start with a heavy weight on your first set and then move down to lighter weights and shorter rest periods as you progress to your fifth set. Workouts such as this are meant to help you develop strength, hypertrophy, and endurance in your legs and throughout your entire body.

Exercise	Sets	Reps	Resistance (%)
Deadlift	5	4,6,8,10,12	Varies
Rest Periods	Varies		

Workout 119
Box Day

Class	Difficulty Level	Time
Mixed	Intermediate	30 minutes

Here, you will use the box jump for a power move in the first exercise by performing five sets of 4 reps with 3 – 4 minutes of rest between sets. Following this, you will use the box jump as an endurance exercise by performing five sets of 20 reps on a shorter box with only 60 seconds of rest between sets. This is a simple workout that exhibits the dual uses of the plyo box: power and endurance. As you fatigue, be sure to focus on landing with your feet squarely on the box. If you feel that you will not be able to land a jump, grab a lower box and try with it rather than forcing it and missing the box.

Exercise	Sets	Reps	Resistance
High Box Jump	5	4	BW
Low Box Jump	5	20	BW
Rest Periods	3-4 minutes, 60 seconds		

63

Workout 120
Machine Wheels

Class	Difficulty Level	Time
Mixed	Advanced	30 minutes

This is a machine dominated workout that starts with a fairly heavy leg press and then progresses to a smith machine lunge. To perform a smith machine lunge, load the smith machine with a relatively light weight and place a plyo box a few feet behind the bar. Begin with your feet shoulder width apart, move your left foot back, and place it onto the plyo box with the balls of your foot making contact with the flat portion of the box. With the bar across your shoulders in a squat position, un-rack the bar and perform a one leg squat. Be sure to keep your chest out, back flat, and eyes looking straight ahead throughout this lift. After this exercise, perform a super-set of leg curls and leg extensions, resting only as long as necessary between sets.

Exercise	Sets	Reps	Resistance (%)
Leg Press	3	6	85
Smith Squat/Lunge	3	8 (Each Leg)	80
Leg Curl	2	12	65
Leg Extension	2	12	65
Rest Periods	Varies		

Workout 121
Last Leg Day

Class	Difficulty Level	Time
Mixed	Advanced	30 minutes

If you only have 30 minutes to get in and out of the gym, this is an excellent go-to lower body workout. The set and rep scheme here will help you to build strength and size throughout your entire body, as heavy, compound movements such as the squat and deadlift can boost more testosterone and growth hormone than exercises that work smaller muscle groups (10).

Exercise	Sets	Reps	Resistance (%)
Squat	3	10	70
Deadlift	3	5	80
Rest Periods	Varies		

Chapter 5

Arm Workouts

I'm not going to lie; biceps and triceps days are not very popular right now. It seems that trainers have decided that because these muscle groups are smaller and are thought of as stereotypical "beach" muscles that training them is pointless. I beg to differ. I believe that, although you certainly can burn more calories and build more muscle by concentrating on larger muscle groups, there is still merit to training the smaller muscles as well because they contribute on each and every lift, as well as in daily activities. There are several ways to approach training the arms; some people like to complete a few sets of the dominate arm muscle after working a larger muscle group i.e. completing a couple of biceps exercises after training your back. Because the biceps are actually performing a great deal of the pulling movements on back exercises such as pull-ups and rows, they are already fatigued at the end of a workout. Completing a few sets of biceps exercises at the end of the workout will help to stimulate growth in these smaller muscles. The same goes for the triceps following a chest or shoulder workout. Another approach to arm training is to work both the biceps and triceps muscles on their own separate day. You could train biceps first, then triceps, or alternate between the two. Because the muscles of the arms are smaller, they do require a bit of a different approach than training larger the muscle groups. For instance, training for power in the arms is very difficult because traditional power exercises such as the clean and jerk or the snatch require large groups of muscles rather than concentration of small muscles. Therefore, this chapter does not include a power section and instead has a larger muscle building section, as we all know that this is what the people want anyway. A good warmup on arm day will include a light exercise that targets the muscle group that you will be targeting in the workout. Try light cable curls and cable press-downs prior to the beginning of your workout.

Arms: Strength Workouts

Workout 122
Strong Bi's

Class	Difficulty Level	Time
Strength	Beginner	30 minutes

Begin this biceps workout with a heavy straight bar curl with a weight that is challenging but with which you can complete 6 reps with good form. Next, move on to dumbbell hammer curls, an excellent exercise to work the biceps as well as the smaller muscles that make up the forearm. Perform three sets of 8 reps with each arm in an alternating fashion. Last, complete a reverse curl with a fixed barbell. This exercise will place even more of an emphasis on the forearms and will help to develop greater grip strength.

Exercise	Sets	Reps	Resistance (%)
Straight Bar Curl	3	6	85
Hammer Curl	3	8	80
Fixed Reverse Curl	3	8	80
Rest Periods		90 seconds	

Workout 123
Strong Chin

Class	Difficulty Level	Time
Strength	Beginner	30 minutes

Begin this workout with two sets each of chin-ups, EZ bar curls, and standing dumbbell curls. To perform the smith drag curl, place a moderate amount of weight on the smith machine and perform a curl while keeping the bar against your stomach until it reaches the bottom portion of your chest. Slowly lower the weight back down in the same fashion, and you have completed 1 rep.

Exercise	Sets	Reps	Resistance (%)
Chin Up	2	6	BW
EZ Bar Curl	2	6	85
Dumbbell Curl	2	8	80
Smith Drag Curl	2	10	70
Rest Periods		90 seconds	

Workout 124
Functional Tri's

Class	Difficulty Level	Time
Strength	Intermediate	25 minutes

Who says arm training can't be functional? The focus of this workout will be on your triceps, but you will certainly be getting a great overall workout, as each of these exercises requires stabilization and assistance from multiple muscle groups. Begin with weighted dips on a parallel dip machine, followed by suspension band bodyweight triceps presses, and narrow push-ups.

Exercise	Sets	Reps	Resistance (%)
Weighted Dips	3	8	85
Band Triceps Press	3	8	80
Narrow Push-ups	3	8	BW
Rest Periods		90 seconds	

Workout 125
Tri Strength

Class	Difficulty Level	Time
Strength	Intermediate	30 minutes

Notice that the exercise order in this workout indicates that complex multi-joint exercises are performed first followed by single joint exercises. This is the optimal order of exercises for both larger and smaller body parts because it allows you to perform exercises that require stabilization from a higher number of muscles while you are less fatigued. A key exception to this rule of thumb is if you want to use a single joint exercise immediately prior to a multi-joint exercise in order to pre-exhaust a muscle. An example of this would be performing a cable rope press down immediately prior to performing close grip push-ups. You will encounter workouts that include a pre-exhaust later in this chapter.

Exercise	Sets	Reps	Resistance (%)
Close Grip Bench	3	8	85
Weighted Dips	3	8	80
Rope Press down	3	8	80
Rest Periods		90 seconds	

Workout 126
Strong Armed

Class	Difficulty Level	Time
Strength	Advanced	30 minutes

This is one of the more difficult arm workouts in this book, and it is meant to be performed in superset fashion, with little to no rest between the chin-ups and the dips. Once you are able to complete the prescribed five sets of 8 reps on each of the moves, you can increase the weight that you are using. If you are a novice lifter, I suggest that you begin with no weight and move up from there.

Exercise	Sets	Reps	Resistance (%)
Weighted Chin-up	5	8	85
Weighted Dip	5	8	Varies
Rest Periods			90 seconds

Workout 127
Alternating Arm Strength

Class	Difficulty Level	Time
Strength	Advanced	30 minutes

This is an excellent arm workout that will hit the biceps and triceps, as well as many of the smaller muscles of the arms. You can perform these sets as either straight sets or supersets with no rest between. Begin with three sets of straight bar curls followed by a behind the head press with a heavy dumbbell. Next, move to three sets of 8 hammer curls with each arm followed by body weight dips on parallel bars. A word of caution: do not perform the straight bar curls in the squat rack; you will be hated.

Exercise	Sets	Reps	Resistance (%)
Straight Bar Curl	3	8	85
Overhead Dumbbell Press	3	8	80
Hammer Curl	3	8	80
Weighted Dips	3	8	50
Rest Periods			90 seconds

Workout 128
Smith Style

Class	Difficulty Level	Time
Strength	Advanced	30 minutes

This workout saves time by allowing you to complete the entire workout on the Smith machine. First, complete inverted smith chin-ups by getting under the smith machine and grasping the bar with an underhand grip. Curl your chest up towards the bar, keeping your elbows in tight, chest up, and back straight. Next, complete three sets of 8 narrow push-ups followed by standing drag curls and close grip presses.

Exercise	Sets	Reps	Resistance (%)
Inverted Smith Chin-up	4	8	BW
Narrow Push-up	4	8	BW
Smith Drag Curl	3	8	80
Close Smith Press	3	8	80
Rest Periods	90 seconds		

Arm Muscle Building Workouts

Workout 129
Bicep Dumbbell Blast

Class	Difficulty Level	Time
Muscle Building	Beginner	25 minutes

All you need is set of dumbbells to complete this workout. Begin with heavy dumbbell hammer curls, alternating each rep between arms. Next, move to dumbbell curls and then switch to dumbbell reverse curls. On all three exercises, including the reverse curls, focus on keeping your elbows in to your sides as you curl the weight up.

Exercise	Sets	Reps	Resistance (%)
Hammer Curl	4	8	70 - 80
Dumbbell Curl	3	10	60 - 70
Reverse Dumbbell Curl	2	12	50 - 60
Rest Periods	60 – 90 seconds		

Workout 130
Tri Time

Class	Difficulty Level	Time
Muscle Building	Beginner	25 minutes

To perform a rope cable extension, place a rope attachment to a cable pulley and stand facing opposite the pulley. Hoist the rope behind your head and bend over with one leg anchored against the cable machine and one in front of you. Keeping your elbows in tight, perform an extension with the rope; focus on using only your triceps to move to the weight. All of the movement on this exercise should take place at the elbow rather than at the shoulder joint. Be sure to keep the natural arch in your back, your chest up, and your head looking straight ahead rather than up or down.

Exercise	Sets	Reps	Resistance (%)
Narrow Push-Up	3	8	BW
Rope Overhead Extension	4	10	70
Cable Press-Down	4	10	70
Rest Periods	60 seconds		

Workout 131
Chin-Up Day

Class	Difficulty Level	Time
Muscle Building	Intermediate	25 minutes

This workout is as simple as it sounds. You will perform one exercise: the chin-up. The goal here is to perform ten sets of 10 chin-ups with 60 seconds of rest in between in each set. Workouts such as this should really be used occasionally in order to avoid over-training and overuse injuries, but it is an excellent option if you are looking to try to spark new growth or just escape the monotony of your current program.

Exercise	Sets	Reps	Resistance (%)
Chin-Up	10	10	BW
Rest Periods	60 seconds		

Workout 132
Pyramid Bi's

Class	Difficulty Level	Time
Muscle Building	Intermediate	30 minutes

Pyramid rep schemes are an excellent way to get a great bang for your buck. This workout entails the use of a pyramid set and rep scheme on each of the three exercises in the workout. Begin with light EZ bar curls for a set of 12 reps. After completing that set, increase the weight by 10 pounds and complete a set of 10 reps. Continue this trend until you finish the fourth set, which calls for 6 reps. Upon finishing this set; begin reducing the weight by 10 pounds on each of the subsequent sets. Perform the next two exercises with the same pyramid scheme.

Exercise	Sets	Reps	Resistance (%)
EZ Bar Curl	7	12,10,8,6,8,10,12	Varies
Cable Bar Curl	5	10,8,6,8,10	Varies
Reverse Cable Bar Curl	5	10,8,6,8,10	Varies
Rest Periods	60 seconds		

71

Workout 133
Cable Arm Day

Class	Difficulty Level	Time
Muscle Building	Intermediate	15 minutes

If you're really pressed for time, this workout can serve as a great way to build muscle on the fly. Begin by performing 8 reps of cable biceps curls immediately followed by 8 reps of triceps press-downs. After two super-sets with the EZ bar attachment, switch to a straight bar attachment for the second superset and then a rope attachment for the third. Alter the weight and reps as shown below.

Exercise	Sets	Reps	Resistance (%)
EZ Cable Curl	4	8	80
EZ Cable Press-down	4	8	80
Straight Bar Cable Curl	3	10	70
Straight Bar Cable Press-Down	3	10	70
Rope Cable Curl	2	12	60
Rope Press-down	2	12	60
Rest Periods	60 seconds		

Workout 134
Triceps Smack down

Class	Difficulty Level	Time
Muscle Building	Intermediate	25 minutes

This is a well-rounded triceps workout that is intended to hit all three heads of that muscle. Begin with weighted dips, followed by dumbbell overhead presses, and finally rope cable press-downs. Complete the second two exercises in the workout as a superset, with no rest between the overhead presses and the cable press-downs.

Exercise	Sets	Reps	Resistance (%)
Dips	4	8	BW
Dumbbell Overhead Press	3	10	70
Rope Press down	3	10	60
Rest Periods	60 seconds		

Workout 135
Huge Tri Day

Class	Difficulty Level	Time
Muscle Building	Advanced	25 minutes

This triceps building workout begins with weighted dips. To stress the triceps more on this move, keep your feet down below the rest of your body and slightly lean back. Both the chest and triceps muscle groups will be worked either way, but you can dictate the extent to which each is impacted by shifting your weight forward and back. Upon finishing the weighted dips, complete four supersets of single dumbbell behind the head extensions and single dumbbell kickbacks.

Exercise	Sets	Reps	Resistance (%)
Weighted Dips	3	8	80
Single Overhead Extension	4	10	70
Single Dumbbell Kick Backs	4	10	70
Narrow Push-ups	3	10	BW
Rest Periods	60 seconds		

Workout 136
Pike's Peaks

Class	Difficulty Level	Time
Muscle Building	Advanced	30 minutes

This workout begins with a heavy, functional bodyweight move and then moves to two single joint exercises. Notice the compound exercises and comparatively shorter rest periods in this workout compared to other arm workouts; this is done to elicit a greater hormonal release throughout the workout (10).

Exercise	Sets	Reps	Resistance (%)
Chin-Ups	5	8	BW
EZ Bar Curls	4	10	80
Hammer Curls	3	12	60
Rest Periods	60 seconds		

Workout 137
Runnin the Strip

Class	Difficulty Level	Time
Muscle Building	Advanced	15 minutes

This workout is comprised of two strip-set exercises and two rack running exercises. First, load an EZ bar with only 10 pound and 5 pound plates until you get to 80% of your 1RM. Complete a set of 6 reps, then immediately remove the outermost weight on each side of the bar and complete 8 reps, and continue lowering the weight until you complete your fourth set, which will be 12 reps. Upon finishing the EZ Bar curls, re-load the weight and perform the same progression with standing EZ Bar extensions. Next, move to the cable machine for the second two exercises. Perform 6 reps of cable curls, and then immediately pull the pin, lower the weight by one or two slots, and perform 8 more reps. Continue until you have finished your fourth set, which will again be 12 reps.

Exercise	Sets	Reps	Resistance (%)
EZ Bar Curl	4	6,8,10,12	Varies
EZ Bar Extension	4	6,8,10,12	Varies
Cable Curl	4	6,8,10,12	Varies
Cable Press-down	4	6,8,10,12	Varies
Rest Periods		60 seconds	

Workout 138
Chin – Up / Narrow Push-up Challenge

Class	Difficulty Level	Time
Muscle Building	Advanced	25 minutes

The goal of this workout is to complete five sets of 10 chin-ups supersetted with narrow push-ups with only 60 seconds of rest between each set. This challenge is one that you can use in a bind when there are no weights around or to simply mix up your current routine. Keep your elbows in tight and use a slightly narrower than shoulder width space between your hands on the narrow push-ups.

Exercise	Sets	Reps	Resistance (%)
Chin-ups	5	10	BW
Narrow Push-ups	5	10	BW
Rest Periods		60 seconds	

Workout 139
Functionally Huge Arms

Class	Difficulty Level	Time
Muscle Building	Advanced	30 minutes

This workout is proof that you can edit and manipulate bodyweight exercises to work your biceps and triceps. I will never understand why it is now considered wrong to train these muscles, but this workout just so you can reap the benefits of arm day and still save face at your gym.

Exercise	Sets	Reps	Resistance (%)
Chin-ups	2	10	BW
Dips	2	10	BW
Inverted Reverse Row	2	10	BW
Narrow Push-up	2	10	BW
Band Curl	2	10	BW
Band Triceps Press	2	10	BW
Rest Periods			60 seconds

Workout 140
All Arms on Deck

Class	Difficulty Level	Time
Muscle Building	Advanced	30 minutes

This all-around arm building workout utilizes functional exercises such as chin-ups and push-ups along with bar exercises like the close grip bench press and straight-bar curl. Notice that the set and rep ranges are similar to those of many of the workouts in this section; the sets are reduced to two per exercise in order to be able to incorporate three exercises for biceps and three for triceps within the 30 minute time period.

Exercise	Sets	Reps	Resistance (%)
Chin Up	2	8	80
Close Grip Bench Press	2	8	80
Straight Bar Curl	2	10	70
Narrow Push-up	2	10	70
Hammer Curl	2	12	60
Rope Press-down	2	12	60
Rest Periods			60 seconds

75

Arms: Endurance Workouts

Workout 141
Narrow Push-up Challenge

Class	Difficulty Level	Time
Endurance	Beginner	30 minutes

This is the same setup as many of the other challenges; here, you will be trying to complete 30 narrow push-ups in as few sets as possible with only 60 seconds of rest between sets. This is an excellent workout to test your anaerobic endurance level using only your bodyweight.

Exercise	Sets	Reps	Resistance (%)
Narrow Push-ups	Varies	30	BW
Rest Periods	60 seconds		

Workout 142
EZ Endurance

Class	Difficulty Level	Time
Endurance	Beginner	15 minutes

If you're a beginner, perform these two exercises as straight sets, which means that you will perform three sets of curls with rest between each set and then perform three sets of extensions with rest between each set. If you are more advanced and ready to add more intensity to the workout, use supersets as a way to push your muscular endurance and to get more blood flow to the arms. This workout could be an excellent burnout, or it could be used as its own workout if you are really crunched for time.

Exercise	Sets	Reps	Resistance (%)
EZ Bar Curls	3	15 - 20	50
EZ Bar Behind the Head Extension	3	15 – 20	50
Rest Periods	60 seconds		

Workout 143
Cable Press-Down Challenge

Class	Difficulty Level	Time
Endurance	Intermediate	15 minutes

This is an excellent finishing exercise following a longer workout, or it can be completed for several sets as one quick endurance workout. Begin by attaching your favorite cable attachment (straight bar, rope, etc…) to the cable apparatus and adjust the weight to a load that will only allow you to complete 4 reps. Complete those 4 reps and then pull the pin and lighten the load by one slot. Complete 6 reps, then immediately pull the pin again, and complete 8. Continue this until you reach the lightest load on the weight stack.

Exercise	Sets	Reps	Resistance (%)
Cable Press-down	Varies	Varies	Varies
Rest Periods	60 seconds		

Workout 144
Chin Up Challenge 2.0

Class	Difficulty Level	Time
Endurance	Intermediate	30 minutes

This challenge will allow you to test the muscular endurance of your biceps and forearms, as well as the muscles in your back such as the lats. The idea here is to perform 100 total chin-ups in as few sets as possible. You may be able to perform 100 chin-ups in one set, or it may take up to fifteen. For instance, you may perform 25 reps in your first set and then fewer in subsequent sets as you fatigue. The key here is to hold rest periods to only 60 seconds between sets. Try to perform the 100 reps in fewer and fewer sets as you progress.

Exercise	Sets	Reps	Resistance (%)
Chin Up	Varies	100	BW
Rest Periods	60 seconds		

Workout 145
Chin-to-Push

Class	Difficulty Level	Time
Endurance	Advanced	25 minutes

This is an excellent workout that will serve to challenge the muscular endurance of your arms with only your body weight. Complete four sets of 15 – 20 chin-ups and four sets of narrow push-ups in a superset fashion, taking no rest between sets.

Exercise	Sets	Reps	Resistance (%)
Chin-ups	4	15 - 20	BW
Narrow Push-ups	4	15 – 20	BW
Rest Periods		60 seconds	

Workout 146
Fixed Flood

Class	Difficulty Level	Time
Endurance	Advanced	30 minutes

This can be used as an excellent burnout at the end of a workout to get extra blood flow to the biceps or as its own workout in a time crunch. Begin by grabbing the heaviest fixed barbell that you can curl with proper form. Curl it twice and then rack it. Immediately grab the next lightest barbell and curl it 4 times. Next, grab the next lightest and curl it 6 times. Continue this until you have curled each of the subsequently lighter fixed barbells, adding 2 reps to each set. Do not rest between each set.

Exercise	Sets	Reps	Resistance (%)
Fixed Barbell Rack Run	Varies	Varies	Varies
Rest Periods		60 seconds	

Arms: Mixed Workouts

Workout 147
Mixed Arms Day

Class	Difficulty Level	Time
Mixed	Beginner	25 minutes

Begin this workout with straight bar curls for four straight sets of 8 reps. Next, perform four sets of 8 narrow push-ups. Be sure to keep the emphasis of this exercise on your triceps by keeping your elbows close to your sides throughout the entire movement. Move to the dumbbell rack for the second two exercises, and complete straight sets of dumbbell hammer curls and dumbbell extensions.

Exercise	Sets	Reps	Resistance (%)
Straight Bar Curl	3	8	80
Narrow Pushups	3	8	BW
Hammer Curl	2	12	65
Dumbbell Triceps Extension	2	12	65
Rest Periods	Varies		

Workout 148
Mixed Bi's One

Class	Difficulty Level	Time
Endurance	Beginner	25 minutes

Perform the first two and second two exercises in this workout back to back with no rest between. Begin with three sets of heavy EZ bar curls, and follow each set immediately with dumbbell hammer curls. Next, move to the cable machine and perform three sets of straight bar cable curls, following each set immediately with reverse cable curls.

Exercise	Sets	Reps	Resistance (%)
EZ Bar Curl	2	8	80
Hammer Curl	2	8	80
Cable Curl	2	12	70
Reverse Cable Curl	2	12	70
Rest Periods	Varies		

Workout 149
Tried True

Class	Difficulty Level	Time
Mixed	Intermediate	25 minutes

If you're looking for an excellent all-around triceps workout, this is the one for you. Although you are concentrating primarily on a smaller muscle group, you can still see better results by beginning with a multi-joint exercise. Start this workout with the close-grip bench press. Go fairly heavy on this exercise and use a competent spotter to help avoid injury.

Exercise	Sets	Reps	Resistance (%)
Close Grip Bench Press	4	6	85
Dips	4	8	BW
Dumbbell Triceps Extension	3	10	70
Cable Press-down	2	12	60
Rest Periods	Varies		

Workout 150
Cables and Function

Class	Difficulty Level	Time
Mixed	Intermediate	25 minutes

Begin this workout by choosing a weight that will allow you to complete 8, but no more than 8 dips. Finding the correct weight to use may take a bit of trial and error, but weighted dips are an excellent way to build muscle in the triceps so it will be worth it. Next, move to narrow push-ups, followed by reverse cable press-downs, and cable press-downs. Once again, rest periods will taper down from longer to shorter duration as you progress through each exercise.

Exercise	Sets	Reps	Resistance (%)
Weighted Dips	4	8	Light Weight
Narrow Push-ups	4	10	BW
Reverse Cable Press-down	2	12	70
Cable Press-down	2	12	60
Rest Periods	Varies		

Workout 151
Super Armed

Class	Difficulty Level	Time
Mixed	Advanced	25 minutes

This workout only requires that you have access to a bench press or cage that will allow you to perform close grip bench presses. Begin by placing a weight on the bar that will allow you to complete 6 reps of close grip bench presses. Once you have completed that set, immediately adjust the weight so that the bar is left with a load that will allow you to complete 6 reps of straight bar curls. Perform those 6 reps and then load the bar with a weight that will allow you to complete 8 reps of close grip bench press, rest two minutes and then move on to the second superset.

Exercise	Sets	Reps	Resistance (%)
Close Grip Bench Press	5	6,8,10,12, 15	Varies
Straight Bar Curl	5	6,8,10,12, 15	Varies
Rest Periods		2 minutes	

Workout 152
Mixed Bi's Two

Class	Difficulty Level	Time
Mixed	Advanced	15 minutes

This mixed biceps workout will take you through strength, muscle building, and endurance phases. A key point to remember on these mixed workouts is that longer rest periods are prescribed for the first exercise, and the rest periods taper down and become progressively shorter as the workout wears on. Here, use two minute rest periods on the first exercise and then work down to 30 second rest periods for the last exercise.

Exercise	Sets	Reps	Resistance (%)
Chin-ups	4	6	BW
Straight Bar Curls	4	8	80
Hammer Curls	3	10	70
Smith Drag Curls	2	12	60
Reverse Cable Curls	2	15	60
Rest Periods		Varies	

Chapter 6

Core Training

Just as Chapter 5 was constructed differently than the bulk of the other chapters, so too is Chapter 6. Here you will find 8 strength building workouts, 8 muscle building workouts, 7 endurance workouts, and 7 mixed workouts. These workouts will require varying types of equipment and implements, and each can be scaled from advanced to novice. While it is possible to increase the power of the core muscles, total body moves like the power clean, squat, and deadlift are more adept at developing power through the core and throughout the entire body. You will be better served to perform those power moves on a separate day than when you perform the following core workouts. Warmups for these exercises could include a light round of cardio and bodyweight exercises such as planks, crunches, and hanging knee raises.

Core: Strength Workouts

Workout 151
Cable Core

Class	Difficulty Level	Time
Strength	Beginner	15 minutes

In order to complete this workout, all you need is a cable cross-over machine and an awesome attitude! Begin with four sets of 8 reps of rope cable crunches with heavy resistance. Next, attach a D-handle to the cable machine and perform 8 cable wood chops to the left followed by 8 to the right. Lastly, attach an ankle strap to the cable crossover and then around your ankles. Lie back flat on the floor with your hands to your side and perform 8 knees to chest reps.

Exercise	Sets	Reps	Resistance (%)
Rope Crunch	3	8	70
Cable Wood Chop	3	8	65
Cable Knees to Chest	3	8	50
Rest Periods	90 seconds		

Workout 152
Decline Strength

Class	Difficulty Level	Time
Strength	Beginner	25 minutes

This workout calls for eight sets of 8 reps of decline crunches. These can be performed with only your body weight, or you can grab either a weight plate or a medicine ball to increase the intensity of the exercise. Do not go all the way back, rather, lean back half way to three – quarters of the way back and then curl your chest toward your knees, focusing on your abdominal muscles rather than your hip-flexors. The hip-flexors will inevitably play a large role in this exercise, which has caused it to lose popularity among many trainers. However, the hip-flexors are part of the body and therefore need to be worked too.

Exercise	Sets	Reps	Resistance (%)
Decline Crunch	5	6 - 8	Varies
Rest Periods	Varies		

Workout 153
Decline Hang

Class	Difficulty Level	Time
Strength	Intermediate	15 minutes

This workout, along with many in the core section, uses only the cable machine. Attach a rope attachment to a cable apparatus and position it about mid-way up the cable machine. Place a decline bench about midway between the two sides of the cable cross-over with the leg stabilizers facing away from the rope attachment. Mount the decline bench and lay back flat; have a partner hand you the rope attachment. With the rope in a similar position to that of a rope cable crunch, curl your chest towards your knees and then let yourself back down, but only halfway. That's one rep. Be careful not to pull the back of your head with your hands or the rope, rather, use your abs to bear the load of curling you up. Perform four sets of 10 hanging leg raises once you finish with the decline cable crunches.

Exercise	Sets	Reps	Resistance (%)
Decline Cable Crunch	4	8	80
Hanging leg raise	4	10	BW
Rest Periods	90 seconds		

Workout 154
Smith Sumo

Class	Difficulty Level	Time
Strength	Intermediate	20 minutes

The first move in this workout is a bit unorthodox, but it should serve to develop strength throughout the core. Start by lying on the ground under a smith machine bar. Extend your arms in the top portion of a bench press, but, instead of lifting the bar with your arms move it with your torso as you curl up with your arms out in front of you holding the bar. Begin by loading a weight that you can handle with ease and then work your up from there once you are more accustomed to the move.

Exercise	Sets	Reps	Resistance (%)
Sumo Deadlift	4	8	80
Smith Curl-Up	4	8	80
Rest Periods	Varies		

Workout 155
Ball Toss / Leg Throw

Class	Difficulty Level	Time
Strength	Intermediate	15 minutes

Perform these two exercises in superset form, with only enough rest as it takes to get from a decline bench to a flat bench. First, mount a decline bench and have your partner toss a relatively heavy medicine ball to you. Catch the ball as you are falling back on the machine and then explosively curl back up and toss the ball back to your partner. That's 1 rep. Perform 10 reps and then immediately lay back on a flat bench with your legs straight out in front of you off of the bench. Secure yourself with your hands grasping the bench behind your head and raise your legs over your hips. Have your friend forcefully push your legs straight down as you try to fight the momentum and keep from allowing your feet to touch the ground. Immediately and explosively bring your feet back up, and your partner will immediately push them back down.

Exercise	Sets	Reps	Resistance
Partner Ball Toss	5	10	Varies
Partner Leg Throw	5	10	BW
Rest Periods		90 seconds	

Workout 156
Standing Core Strength

Class	Difficulty Level	Time
Strength	Intermediate	25 minutes

Begin this workout by attaching a rope to the cable crossover machine and performing four sets of 8 cable crunches while standing. Next, move to standing oblique cable curls; perform four sets of 8 reps before finishing the workout with four sets of 10 bodyweight back extensions to strengthen the lower back.

Exercise	Sets	Reps	Resistance (%)
Cable Crunch	4	8	80
Standing Cable Oblique Crunch	4	8	80
Back Extension	4	10	BW
Rest Periods		90 seconds	

Workout 157
Abstrongables

Class	Difficulty Level	Time
Strength	Advanced	25 minutes

Begin this workout by performing four sets of 8 leg raises, raising a dumbbell straight out in front of you until your legs and back form a 90 degree angle. Next, perform a series of rope cable pulls. Attach a rope to a cable pulley and lower it about two feet off of the floor. Stand facing away from the rope, then bend over and grasp the rope and situate it between your legs. Raise your torso, keeping your chest up, back flat, and arms relatively immobile until you are standing straight up with the rope in front of your hips. That's 1 rep. For the last exercise, grab a 25 pound plate, depending on your strength level, and lie flat on your back on the floor next to it. Lift your legs straight up, forming a 90 degree angle with your legs and torso. Hold the weight plate in front of your chest and face and extend your arms to almost lock out and curl yourself up.

Exercise	Sets	Reps	Resistance (%)
Weighted Leg Raise	4	8	60 - 70
Cable Pull-through	4	8	60 - 70
Plate Raise	4	8	60 - 70
Rest Periods			Varies

Workout 158
Sumo Strongback

Class	Difficulty	Time
Strength	Advanced	30 minutes

The deadlift, and all of the variations of the deadlift are excellent for building strength in the lower back. Begin this workout with three sets of sumo deadlifts followed by the more traditional core exercises listed.

Exercise	Sets	Reps	Resistance (%)
Sumo Deadlift	3	8	75
Rope Cable Crunch	3	8	80
Ab Machine	3	8	80
Med Ball Side to Side	3	16	80
Rest Periods			90 seconds

Core: Muscle Building Workouts

Workout 159
Rope All Day

Class	Difficulty Level	Time
Muscle Building	Beginner	15 minutes

This straightforward cable crunch workout is great to mix things up as a burnout or as a quick hitting core workout. Simply attach a rope to a cable pulley and perform ten sets of 10 rope cable crunches. Use fairly heavy weight for the first few sets and concentrate on squeezing your abs during the concentric portion of the workout.

Exercise	Sets	Reps	Resistance (%)
Rope Cable Crunch	5	10	70
Rest Periods	60 seconds		

Workout 160
Straight Abs

Class	Difficulty Level	Time
Muscle Building	Beginner	25 minutes

This workout features four straight sets of ab exercises. Begin with cable crunches and then move to hanging leg raises. After the leg raises, find an ab machine and perform three sets of 10 crunches. While many trainers shy away from machines in general, especially ab machines, I think that within a larger workout they can be advantageous because they allow you to move more weight with these muscles than is typically possible using body weight exercises only. Finish the workout with three sets of 10 cable wood chops to each side.

Exercise	Sets	Reps	Resistance (%)
Cable Crunch	3	10	70
Ab Machine Crunch	3	10	70
Cable Wood Chops	3	10	70
Rest Periods	60 seconds		

Workout 161
Med Ball Madness

Class	Difficulty Level	Time
Muscle Building	Intermediate	25 minutes

The first exercise here, the medicine ball throw, will target your abs as well as your hip flexors, so it may not be the best exercise to perform on days immediately before or after heavy leg days. The next two exercises in the workout are fairly standard, but the last exercise warrants some explanation. Begin the lying cable crunch by placing the cable handle on the lowest setting on the cable cross machine and attach a rope attachment to it. Lie down on the floor a few feet in front of the cable and anchor your feet to keep them from moving. Grasp the rope behind your head and pull it to the sides of your head. Perform weighted crunches in this position.

Exercise	Sets	Reps	Resistance (%)
Medicine Ball Throw	3	10	5 lbs. – 25 lbs.
Machine Crunch	3	10	70
Hanging Leg Raise	3	10	5 lbs. – 25 lbs.
Laying Cable Crunch	3	10	70
Rest Periods			60 seconds

Workout 162
Drop Set Core

Class	Difficulty Level	Time
Muscle Building	Intermediate	15 minutes

This workout begins with hanging leg raises. Place a dumbbell between your feet and perform 10 hanging leg raises while holding onto the weight. Once you have completed 10, drop the weight and complete and 10 more rep before moving onto the next exercise.

Exercise	Sets	Reps	Resistance (%)
Hanging Leg Raise	2	10	10 – 25 lbs.
Hanging Knee Raise	2	10	BW
Weighted Decline Crunch	2	10	10 – 25 lbs.
Decline Crunch	2	10	BW
Weighted Glute/Ham	2	10	10 – 25 lbs.
Glute Ham	2	10	BW
Rest Periods			90 seconds

Workout 163
Fast

Class	Difficulty Level	Time
Muscle Building	Advanced	30 minutes

Begin this muscle building workout with three straight sets of weighted leg raises to target your abs. Next, move to weighted hyperextensions to target your lower back and then perform three sets of cable wood chops to each side. Finally, finish this workout off with three sets of rope cable crunches which will tax your entire core by applying consistent resistance throughout the movement.

Exercise	Sets	Reps	Resistance (%)
Hanging Leg Raise	3	10	5 lbs. – 25 lbs.
Weighted Back Ext.	3	10	10 lbs. – 25 lbs.
Cable Wood chop	3 (Each Side)	10	20
Rope Cable Crunch	3	10	70
Rest Periods		60 seconds	

Workout 164
Decline Ab Day

Class	Difficulty Level	Time
Muscle Building	Advanced	25 minutes

This is another challenging but simple workout. Perform ten sets of 10 weighted decline crunches. Use heavier weight than you typically would on a decline crunch for 20 or 25 reps, as you are only performing half as many reps in each set here. Further, keep in mind that your hip flexors and quads are likely to become exhausted during this exercise, as they must stabilize throughout the workout.

Exercise	Sets	Reps	Resistance (%)
Weighted Decline Crunch	10	10	70
Rest Periods		60 seconds	

Workout 165
Washboard

Class	Difficulty Level	Time
Muscle Building	Advanced	30 minutes

Begin this workout by mounting the bench and make sure that your legs are securely locked into place; perform the eccentric portion of the move by lying back on the bench. Once your back is flush with the bench, reach back and grab the medicine ball. In one fluid motion, grab the ball and bring it in front of your head as you perform the concentric portion of the lift. Once you reach the top, perform the same move again, this time bringing the ball over your head as you lay back. Place the ball on the floor and perform the upward portion of the lift with no weight and subsequently lie back down and pick the ball up again.

Exercise	Sets	Reps	Resistance (%)
Decline Ball Pickup	3	10	10 – 25 lbs.
Cable Wood Chops	3	10	70
Lying Leg Raise	3	10	BW
Weighted Glute/Ham	3	10	10 – 25 lbs.
Rest Periods			90 seconds

Workout 166
Stair Down Abs

Class	Difficulty Level	Time
Muscle Building	Advanced	20 minutes

Begin by placing the weight on your 12 rep max and complete 12 reps. Rest 30 seconds, increase the weight slightly and then perform 10 reps. To perform the second exercise in this workout, lower the cable attachment to the bottom setting and attach the ankle straps (or D handles) to the cable machine. Lie flat on your back and grasp the other side of the cable machine to anchor yourself down. Bring your knees to your chest under control and then slowly extend them back out.

Exercise	Sets	Reps	Resistance (%)
Cable Crunch	4	12,10,8,6	Varies
Lying Cable Leg Curl	4	12,10,8,6	Varies
Cable Wood Chops	4	12,10,8,6	Varies
Rest Periods			60 seconds

Core: Endurance Workouts

Workout 167
Living Room Abs

Class	Difficulty Level	Time
Endurance	Beginner	20 minutes

You can work on that mid-section with workouts that require nothing more than your body. Begin with a plank rotation, which entails performing middle, left, and right side planks in 10, 15 or 30 second intervals with no rest between. Next, perform bicycle crunches: lie back and place your hands behind your head and repetitively bring your right elbow to your left knee and vice versa. Lastly, lay back with your knees bent in front of you. Move your body side to side and touch your heels with your hands as you go back and forth. These exercises can be performed as straight sets if you are a beginner or as a superset if you are more advanced.

Exercise	Sets	Reps	Resistance (%)
Plank Rotation	3	2 minutes	BW
Bicycle Crunch	3	50	BW
Fingers to Heels	3	50	BW
Rest Periods	60 seconds		

Workout 168
Walk the Plank

Class	Difficulty Level	Time
Endurance	Beginner	15 minutes

Planks are an excellent exercise because they work the core which stabilizes and maintains posture in the upper body. Begin each set with 30 seconds of a neutral or "middle" plank, then immediately rotate onto your right forearm and place your left hand on your left hip. Hold this pose for 30 seconds then switch to the right for 30 seconds. Finish with 30 seconds back to the middle. If you are unable to hold the planks for 30 seconds, lower each interval time to 10 - 15 seconds and work your way up.

Exercise	Sets	Reps	Resistance (%)
Plank Rotation	3	2 minutes	BW
Rest Periods	60 seconds		

Workout 169
Band Interval

Class	Difficulty Level	Time
Endurance	Intermediate	15 minutes

To perform "The Runner," get into a push-up position in front of a suspension band. Place one foot into the stirrup behind you. While bracing yourself, place your other foot into the other stirrup. Now, get into a push-up position and bring your right knee to your chest followed immediately by your left knee, as if you are running. Once you have finished 20 of these total, move immediately to medicine ball side to sides, hanging leg raises, and bodyweight crunches in superset fashion.

Exercise	Sets	Reps	Resistance (%)
The Runner	3	20	70
Medicine Ball Side to Side	3	20	BW
Hanging Leg Raise	3	20	50
Bodyweight Crunch	3	50	BW
Rest Periods			60 seconds

Workout 170
100's

Class	Difficulty Level	Time
Endurance	Intermediate	25 minutes

This is a quick, straightforward workout that you can perform in as little as 10 – 15 minutes. Begin by performing 100 hanging leg raises in as few sets as possible to reach 100 reps. If you are a bit more advanced you may be able to complete 100 reps in as few as one or two sets, but if not, it may take four or five sets. Complete the bicycle crunches, sit ups, and toe touches using the same method.

Exercise	Sets	Reps	Resistance (%)
Hanging Leg Raises	1	100	BW
Bicycle Crunch	1	100	BW
Sit Up	1	100	BW
Toe Touches	1	100	BW
Rest Periods			60 seconds

Workout 171
Partner Core Work

Class	Difficulty Level	Time
Endurance	Advanced	15 minutes

This is a quick endurance core workout that would serve as a nice cap to a larger workout, or it can be completed on its own. Begin with four straight sets of partner leg throws and then complete four straight sets of partner medicine ball tosses on a decline bench. While the abs are all one unit, you will feel more of a burn in the lower portion of your abs on the leg throws and more of a burn in the upper portion of the abs on the medicine ball tosses. This is result of both the angles that you will be working in and the other muscles that come into play during each exercise.

Exercise	Sets	Reps	Resistance (%)
Leg Throw	4	25	BW
Ball Toss	4	25	5 – 10 lbs.
Rest Periods			60 seconds

Workout 172
Cable Endurance

Class	Difficulty Level	Time
Endurance	Advanced	15 minutes

This workout can be completed in 10 to 15 minutes if you don't stop and talk to people. Begin with a hanging side to side knee raise. Here, grab the pull-up bars on a cable machine and bring your knees up to 90 degrees. Bend to the right, bringing your hips up to that side. Next, bend to the left, bringing your hips to that side. That's one rep. After completing two sets of 25 reps, complete two sets of 25 reps of hanging knee raises to the front. From there, move to rope cable crunches followed by cable wood chops.

Exercise	Sets	Reps	Resistance (%)
Side to Side Knee Raise	2	25	BW
Straight Knee Raise	2	25	BW
Rope Cable Crunch	2	25	40
Cable Wood Chop	2	25	40
Rest Periods			60 seconds

Workout 173
Raise and Rope

Class	Difficulty Level	Time
Endurance	Advanced	10 minutes

This is a workout that can be completed as a single workout or as a burnout at the end of another workout. The idea here is to perform your max number of leg raises when you are fresh followed immediately by an equal number of rope cable crunches. Next, complete slightly fewer leg raises followed immediately by that same amount of rope cable crunches, all with no rest between sets. The number of reps to complete in each set decreases as you fatigue, which will help you to finish the workout. You will not rest at any point in this workout.

Exercise	Sets	Reps	Resistance (%)
Leg Raise	5	25, 20, 15, 10, 5	BW
Rope Cable Crunch	5	25, 20, 15, 10, 5	5 – 10 lbs.
Rest Periods			0 seconds

Core: Mixed Workouts

Workout 174
Roped

Class	Difficulty Level	Time
Mixed	Beginner	10 minutes

You can complete this workout using straight sets if you are a beginner or supersets if you are more advanced. To complete the workout with supersets, begin with 10 reps of fairly heavy cable crunches followed immediately by 10 reps of cable wood chops to each side. As you progress through the reps, lighten the load and decrease the rest periods. This workout should only take around 10 minutes.

Exercise	Sets	Reps	Resistance (%)
Rope Cable Crunch	5	10, 12, 15, 12, 10	Varies
Cable Wood Chop	5	10, 12, 15, 12, 10	Varies
Rest Periods		Varies	

Workout 175
Cored

Class	Difficulty Level	Time
Mixed	Beginner	25 minutes

This workout can either be performed as an interval or in straight sets with rest between each set and exercise. Begin by placing an ab ball on the floor and form a plank position with your feet on the ball, keeping your arms straight but not locked out, your chest up, and your back flat. Bring your right knee up to your chest and then rapidly place it back in the starting position. Next, bring your left knee to your chest then place it back to the start position. That's one rep. Complete two sets of 6 reps and then move to the ab roller, bicycle crunches, and toe touches.

Exercise	Sets	Reps	Resistance (%)
Ab Ball Knees to Chest	2	6	BW
Ab roller	2	8	BW
Bicycle Crunches	3	20	BW
Toe Touch	3	20	BW
Rest Periods		90 seconds	

Workout 176
Mixed Core Circuit

Class	Difficulty Level	Time
Mixed	Intermediate	15 minutes

This circuit alternates a weighted dynamic core move with a stationary bodyweight exercise in order to tax both the fast twitch and slow twitch muscle fibers of the core. Perform the first set of each exercise in a circuit fashion, then rest 90 seconds and complete the circuit a second time. This workout should only take 15 to 20 minutes, depending on how long you flex your abs in the mirror.

Exercise	Sets	Reps	Resistance (%)
Cable Wood Chop	2	10	70
Plank	2	30 seconds	BW
Cable Wood Chop	2	10	60
Left Side Plank	2	30 seconds	BW
Cable Wood Chop	2	10	50
Right Side Plank	2	30 seconds	BW
Rest Periods		90 seconds	

Workout 177
Weighted Core

Class	Difficulty Level	Time
Mixed	Intermediate	25 minutes

This workout places an emphasis on using resistance to train the core muscles of the abs and the muscles of the lower back. Begin with weighted decline crunches followed by weighted leg raises, weighted glute/ham raises, and a plank rotation. Like many of the other workouts in this section, this is a great overall core workout that can be done on its own or as a part of a larger workout.

Exercise	Sets	Reps	Resistance (%)
Weighted Decline Crunch	3	10	50
Weighted Leg Raise	3	10	50
Weighted Glute/Ham	3	10	50
Plank Rotation	3	2 minutes	BW
Rest Periods		90 seconds	

96

Workout 178
Declining Core

Class	Difficulty Level	Time
Mixed	Advanced	25 minutes

This workout will center on the decline bench exclusively. Perform this workout using straight sets and with a partner. Begin by completing three sets of 10 decline medicine ball tosses. Next, grab a light dumbbell and lean back about halfway on the decline bench. Hold out the dumbbell with both hands and move it from one side to the other under control. Next, take that same dumbbell and perform three sets of 12 crunches followed by three sets of 12 non-weighted crunches.

Exercise	Sets	Reps	Resistance (%)
Decline Medicine Ball Toss	3	10	60
Decline Dumbbell Side Rotation	3	12	60
Decline Dumbbell Crunch	3	12	760
Decline BW Crunch	3	20	BW
Rest Periods			90 seconds

Workout 179
Dead Core

Class	Difficulty Level	Time
Mixed	Advanced	10 minutes

The deadlift is one of the premier exercises for building power and strength throughout the entire body, including the core. Even if you have strong legs and a strong upper body, your overall strength, power, and explosiveness will be lacking if you do not have a strong core. After completing three sets of heavy deadlifts, perform the three assistance moves below to help build your core.

Exercise	Sets	Reps	Resistance (%)
Deadlift	3	5	70
Rope Cable Crunch	3	8	70
Hanging Leg Raise	3	12	60
Plank Rotation	1	3 minutes	BW
Rest Periods			90 seconds

Workout 180
Hang Man

Class	Difficulty Level	Time
Mixed	Advanced	25 minutes

This workout can be performed in straight sets or as a circuit. The exercises are organized by the most difficult to least difficult, which is reflected by the rep schemes. Begin with weighted hanging leg raises followed by weighted hanging knee raises, hanging leg raises without weight, hanging knee raises without weight, and side to side knee raises.

Exercise	Sets	Reps	Resistance (%)
Weighted Hanging Leg Lift	3	8	5 – 25 lbs.
Weighted Hanging Knee Lift	3	10	5 – 25 lbs.
Hanging Leg Lift	3	12	BW
Hanging Knee Lift	3	12	BW
Hanging Side to Side Knee Lift	3	12	BW
Rest Periods			90 seconds

Chapter 7

High Intensity Interval Workouts

This chapter will provide 30 HIIT or High Intensity Interval Training workouts. These workouts can be described as a series of back to back exercises that can feature cardio, strength training or both, with relatively little rest between sets. The American College of Sports Medicine rated HIIT as the #1 exercise trend in the United States in 2014 (1). There is good reason for the recent popularity in HIIT; as it is purported to be one of the best methods to burn body fat and to build lean muscle. As you flip through this chapter you should notice that most of these workouts are built around body weight exercises and short sprint cycles. This is because from a safety standpoint, it is best to perform Olympic and other dynamic lifts with plenty of rest between each set. Instead of using moves like the squat, deadlift, power clean, or bench press, you will primarily be using strict pull-ups, push-ups, barbell curls, ab crunches, and cable / TRX exercises. This chapter is unique in that it is not divided into power, strength, hypertrophy, etc… instead, it is simply a collection of 30 HIIT workouts. Also note that there are many more intermediate and advanced workouts than there are beginner workouts in this chapter, as high intensity interval training by its very nature is not really meant for beginners. While there are a couple of workouts that I felt comfortable designating as for beginners, there are not many. Before you perform a HIIT workout, you should consult with a certified fitness professional such as a strength coach or exercise physiologist. As with the other chapters, the time for completion will vary depending on many factors, including warmup and cool down time. Prior to beginning any of these workouts complete a thorough warmup that consists first of slow, steady movement, and later more dynamic explosive movements. A good warmup for a HIIT day would be to spend 5 – 10 minutes on the treadmill, gradually increasing the intensity each minute. After that, jump rope for 2 – 3 minutes or complete a series of jumping jacks. Cool downs are just as important as warmups following a HIIT session. To cool down, begin running on the treadmill at a relatively fast pace and incrementally decrease the intensity each minute for 5 – 10 minutes.

Workout 181
Track Ladder

Class	Difficulty Level	Time
HIIT	Beginner	15 minutes

Many gyms now have core sections next to their running tracks, so workouts like this become more plausible. Begin by jogging 1 lap as a warm-up and then pick up the pace for the first "official" lap. Immediately after you complete 1 lap, go to the core section and complete a plank for 1 minute. After your plank, run 2 more laps on the track followed by a plank on your right side. Complete the 3 lap run, left side plank, and the 4 lap run and then cool down with a light jog around the track.

Exercise	Sets	Reps (Laps)	Resistance
Track Run	Laps	1	BW
Plank (Neutral)	30 Seconds		BW
Track Run	Laps	2	BW
Plank (Right Side)	30 Seconds		BW
Track Run	Laps	3	BW
Plank (Left Side)	30 Seconds		BW
Track Run	Laps	4	BW
Rest Periods	60 seconds between sets		

Workout 182
Hotel Room HIIT

Class	Difficulty Level	Time
HIIT	Beginner	15 minutes

Complete two rounds of the following workout: begin with 15 burpees and then progress to 30 crunches and 50 lying toe touches. Extend the number of sets or reps to increase the challenge, or throw in a set or two of planks to round out the workout if you have time. This is a quick hitting workout that can be completed after an upper body workout, or it on its own as a quick calorie burner.

Exercise	Sets	Reps	Resistance
Burpees	2	15	BW
Crunches	2	30	BW
Toe Touch	2	50	BW
Rest Periods	2 minutes		

Workout 183
HIIT the Beach

Class	Difficulty Level	Time
HIIT	Intermediate	20 minutes

Running in the sand is a great way to develop the muscles of the lower legs and really to challenge the entire body. However, this workout can be completed anywhere that you have a relatively open and flat area to run. Find a clear, open spot on the beach and draw a line in the sand with your foot. Next, walk roughly 40 yards in a straight line and draw another line in the sand. This is your starting point. Assume a push-up position and perform 5 plyo-push-ups. On the fifth push-up, jump up and sprint to the first line that you drew. Upon reaching that line, get down and perform 10 regular push-ups. That's one set.

Exercise	Sets	Reps	Resistance (%)
Plyo-Pushups	5	5	BW
40 Yard Dash	5	-	BW
Pushups	5	10	BW
Rest Periods		60 seconds between sets	

Workout 184
Cable Machine Madness

Class	Difficulty Level	Time
HIIT	Intermediate	15 minutes

This interval workout can be completed at either a standard cable cross-over machine or a functional cable machine. Perform 10 pull-ups (or as many as you can up to 10) first while you are fresh and then immediately perform 10 hanging leg raises. After finishing the leg raises, immediately drop to the floor and perform 10 push-ups followed immediately by 10 rope cable crunches. This workout is a great way to jack up your heart rate without doing any traditional cardio.

Exercise	Sets	Reps	Resistance (%)
Wide Grip Pull-up	5	10	BW
Hanging Leg Raise	5	10	BW
Push-ups	5	10	BW
Rope Cable Crunch	5	10	50
Rest Periods		90 seconds between intervals	

Workout 185
Chest Back HIIT

Class	Difficulty Level	Time
HIIT	Intermediate	15 minutes

After a proper warm-up, begin by completing a set of 10 wide grip pull-ups. Next, begin jogging on a track; as you turn the corner of the track begin to pick up your pace and then sprint the length of the next piece of the track. Once you turn the corner again, slow down to a jog and then walk back to the chin-up / dip machine for your first set of dips.

Exercise	Sets	Reps	Resistance (%)
Wide Grip Pull-up	1	10	BW
Jog/Sprint/Jog	1	-	BW
Bodyweight Dip	1	10	BW
Jog/Sprint/Jog	1	-	BW
Wide Pull-up	1	10	BW
Jog/Sprint/Jog	1	-	BW
Bodyweight Dip	1	10	BW
Rest Periods	30 seconds between sets		

Workout 186
Suspension Meets HIIT

Class	Difficulty Level	Time
HIIT	Intermediate	15 minutes

This workout is meant to be performed as an interval with very little to no rest in between each exercise. Begin with suspension chest presses and then immediately turn the opposite direction and perform suspension inverted rows. After these, move over to a high box and perform 5 box jumps followed by 15 burpees. That's one interval. Complete five of these intervals.

Exercise	Sets	Reps	Resistance (%)
Suspension Chest Press	5	10	BW
Suspension Inverted Row	5	10	BW
Box Jump	5	5	BW
Burpees	5	15	BW
Rest Periods			60 seconds

Workout 187
Hoop Dreams

Class	Difficulty Level	Time
HIIT	Intermediate	15 minutes

Sometimes the best thing to do in the gym is to mix it up and incorporate something you just really enjoy doing. Begin this workout with a game of one on one against yourself. Here's how to play: Begin with a foul shot; if you make it, you get one point. If you miss it, the "other team" gets two points. Grab the rebound and shoot again. Regardless of whether you make the basket, the ball can only bounce twice on the rebound. If it bounces more than twice on the rebound, you have to immediately perform 10 push-ups for each extra bounce of the ball. Regardless of where the ball lands on the rebound, you only get two dribbles before you have to shoot again. Play to ten and move to the baseline for suicides.

Exercise	Sets	Reps	Resistance (%)
U v U	1	-	BW
Suicide	2	-	BW
Jump Rope	2	50	BW
Suicide	1	-	BW
Rest Periods	60 seconds		

Workout 188
Pull Push

Class	Difficulty Level	Time
HIIT	Intermediate	10 minutes

This is a burnout that can be completed as a single workout or at the end of another workout. The idea here is to perform your max number of pull-ups followed immediately by an equal number of push-ups and then to complete a slightly less amount of pull-ups followed immediately by that same amount of push-ups, all with no rest between sets. In summary, you will complete five sets of pull-ups and 5 sets of push-ups with no rest.

Exercise	Sets	Reps	Resistance (%)
Pull-up	5	15, 12, 10, 8, 5	BW
Push-up	5	15, 12, 10, 8, 5	BW
Rest Periods	0 seconds		

Workout 189
HIITastic

Class	Difficulty Level	Time
HIIT	Intermediate	20 minutes

This is another functional, high intensity workout that features bodyweight moves only. Perform each of these exercises in back to back fashion with no rest between exercises. Start with bodyweight dips, then move immediately to inverted rows in a rack, on a smith machine or using suspension bands, and finish with a plank rotation in which you spend 15 seconds each on neutral, right, and left planks.

Exercise	Sets	Reps	Resistance (%)
Dip	5	10	BW
Inverted Row	5	10	BW
Plank Rotation	5	1 minute	BW
Rest Periods		30 seconds	

Workout 190
Pull Push Pyramid

Class	Difficulty Level	Time
HIIT	Intermediate	15 minutes

This is an excellent HIIT workout that will challenge you both aerobically and anaerobically. Perform the prescribed pull-ups and push-ups with no rest between each set. Begin with a single pull-up and then immediately drop and perform 1 push-up. Stand up and immediately perform 2 pull-ups again followed immediately by 2 push-ups. Next, bounce back up and perform 3 pull-ups followed immediately by 3 push-ups. Now work your way back down, beginning with 2 pull-ups and 2 push-ups followed by 1 pull-up and 1 push-up. Rest 3 minutes then begin the interval again.

Exercise	Sets	Reps	Resistance (%)
1 Pull-up / 1 Push-up	3	1	BW
2 Pull-ups / 2 Push-ups	3	1	BW
3 Pull-ups / 3 Push-ups	3	2	BW
2 Pull-ups / 2 Push-ups	3	2	BW
1 Pull-ups / 1 Push-ups	3	3	BW
Rest Periods		2 minutes	

Workout 191
Rock Solid

Class	Difficulty Level	Time
HIIT	Advanced	30 minutes

This workout is named after the movie that won the award for the greatest movie ever... Rocky IV. I could go on for days about the reasons why Rocky IV is the greatest movie ever, but there's no time for that now. This workout is awesome as well, as it will push you with a mix of boxing moves, agility drills, and strength training. Begin this workout with either a car push or a sled push. Bring a friend along to drive if you use the car. Perform the first exercise in straight set fashion, and then complete the last three exercises as an interval.

Exercise	Sets	Reps	Resistance (%)
Sled Push	3	40 Yards	Heavy
Side to side pull-up	4	10	BW
Jump Rope	4	100	BW
Heavy Bag	4	1 min.	BW
Rest Periods		2 minutes	

Workout 192
Functional Fitness

Class	Difficulty Level	Time
HIIT	Advanced	20 minutes

This is a very difficult interval that requires only a straight bar for muscle-ups and pull-ups. Begin each interval with as many muscle ups as you can perform up to 3. Immediately following the muscle-ups, perform 5 explosive pull-ups in which your hands come off of the bar at the top and then catch the bar during your descent. Upon completion of the fifth rep, immediately perform 10 leg raises and then drop and complete 5 clap push-ups.

Exercise	Sets	Reps	Resistance (%)
Bar Muscle-ups	3	3	BW
Plyo Pull-ups	3	5	BW
Leg Raises	3	10	BW
Plyo Push-ups	3	5	BW
Rest Periods		2 minutes	

Workout 193
Animal

Class	Difficulty Level	Time
HIIT	Advanced	20 minutes

This workout should be fairly quick, as the setup time is minimal. Load a bar with a weight with which you could typically perform at least 10 clean and jerks. Begin by performing 4 hang-cleans followed immediately by 4 jerks, 4 upright rows, and 4 shrugs. You will be using the same bar and same weight on all four of these exercises and will not rest between exercises. Once you finish the shrugs, drop the barbell and perform 4 burpees. This workout is not about using heavy weight; rather, the focus should stay on using good form and rapidly increasing your heart rate ... which will happen.

Exercise	Sets	Reps	Resistance (%)
Hang Clean	4	4	50
Jerk	4	4	50
Upright Row	4	4	50
Shrug	4	4	50
Burpees	4	4	BW
Rest Periods		2 minutes	

Workout 194
Pull Push Plank

Class	Difficulty Level	Time
HIIT	Advanced	20 minutes

This simple workout can be performed with access only to a straight bar. Begin the circuit by performing 10 pull-ups, followed immediately by 10 push-ups, and finally a plank for 30 seconds. Rest one minute and then perform the interval four more times, with one minute of rest between each.

Exercise	Sets	Reps	Resistance (%)
Pull-up	5	10	BW
Push-up	5	10	BW
Plank	5	1 minutes	BW
Rest Periods		60 - 90 seconds	

106

Workout 195
Cardio Incorporated

Class	Difficulty Level	Time
HIIT	Advanced	30 minutes

Begin this workout with a one mile run, either on a track, treadmill, or outside, and then move immediately into the interval. Once you have completed three rounds of the interval, complete a second one mile run to finish the workout.

Exercise	Sets	Reps	Resistance
1 Mile Run	1	-	BW
Jump Squats	3	5	BW
Plyo Pushups	3	10	BW
Burpees	3	15	BW
1 Mile Run	1	-	BW
Rest Periods	90 seconds		

Workout 196
Lapped

Class	Difficulty Level	Time
HIIT	Advanced	30 minutes

Begin this workout with a one minute plank rotation followed immediately by a sprint around the track at your highest sustainable intensity for 1 lap. Upon completing that fast lap, slow to 65 – 75% intensity and run two more laps followed by 3 laps of a jog. Next, make your way back to the side and complete a second plank rotation. Continue in the same way.

Exercise	Sets	Reps	Resistance (%)
Plank Rotation	1	1 minutes	BW
1 Lap	Sprint		50%
2 Laps	Run		70%
3 Laps	Jog		50%
Plank Rotation	1	1 minutes	BW
3 Laps	Jog		50%
2 Laps	Run		70%
1 Lap	Sprint		90%
Plank Rotation	1	1 minutes	BW
Rest Periods	90 seconds		

Workout 197
Plyo Drop

Class	Difficulty Level	Time
HIIT	Advanced	30 minutes

This workout is comprised of explosive versions of an exercise followed immediately by its traditional version. Begin by completing three sets of 5 explosive pull-ups followed immediately by 10 normal rep speed pull-ups. Next, run 1 lap on a track and then get into position for push-ups. Perform three sets of 5 explosive push-ups followed immediately by normal rep speed push-ups. Normal rep speed is considered taking two seconds on both the eccentric and concentric portions of the lift. Finish the workout with another quick run.

Exercise	Sets	Reps	Resistance (%)
Plyo Pull-up	3	5	BW
Pull-up	3	10	BW
1 Lap Run	1	-	70
Plyo Pushup	3	5	BW
Pushup	3	10	BW
1 Lap Run	1	-	70
Rest Periods	60 seconds		

Workout 198
The Mile

Class	Difficulty Level	Time
HIIT	Advanced	15 minutes

To complete this workout, you need either a running track or a treadmill. Although you are running a mile, you should be on the verge of anaerobic rather than aerobic energy because you will be pushing to beat your best previous time (6).

Exercise	Sets	Reps	Resistance (%)
1 Mile Run	For Time		BW
Rest Periods	-		

Workout 199
HIIT Don't Quit

Class	Difficulty Level	Time
HIIT	Advanced	15 minutes

If you stick to the prescribed intensities, this high intensity workout is far more brutal than it looks on paper. Begin with one set of challenging box jumps followed immediately by a single lap run at what you perceive as 90% intensity. Continue in this manner while resting only 20 seconds between each set.

Exercise	Sets	Reps	Resistance (%)
Box Jump	1	5	BW
1 Lap Run	-	-	90
Pull-up	1	20	BW
2 Lap Run	-	-	80
Push-up	1	20	BW
3 Lap Run	-	-	70
Pull-up	1	15	BW
4 Lap Run	-	-	60
Push-up	1	15	BW
Rest Periods	20 seconds		

Workout 200
Bodyweight Blast

Class	Difficulty Level	Time
HIIT	Advanced	25 minutes

This workout will jack your heart rate by using a combination of bodyweight moves that target your entire body. Begin by performing 20 bodyweight jump squats. Follow this up immediately with 20 push-ups and 20 chin-ups. Rest for two minutes and then complete another round.

Exercise	Sets	Reps	Resistance (%)
Jump Squat	4	20	BW
Push-up	4	20	BW
Chin-Up	4	20	BW
Rest Periods	2 minutes		

Workout 201
HIIT The Pool

Class	Difficulty Level	Time
HIIT	Advanced	15 minutes

Begin this workout with 2 down and back laps at a 60-70% intensity pace. Next, make your way over to the shallow end of the pool and run 2 down and back laps from one side of the shallow end to the other. From here, rest briefly then swim all out for one down and back. Finish the workout with 2 more runs in the shallow end and 2 laps at your own pace.

Exercise	Sets	Reps	Resistance (%)
Lap Swim	2 Laps		BW
Pool Run	2 Laps		BW
Swim Sprint	Sprint Down and Back		BW
Pool Run	2 Laps		BW
Lap Swim	2 Laps		BW
Rest Periods	90 seconds		

Workout 202
The Stairs

Class	Difficulty Level	Time
HIIT	Advanced	15 minutes

The goal here is to mix a dynamic form of cardio with functional explosive moves in a non-stop fashion in order to improve aerobic endurance as well as muscular endurance. Find a flight of stairs that spans 2 or 3 floors and run up the stairs. Once you reach the top, perform 5 box jumps, followed immediately by one minute of jump roping, and 25 pushups. Run back down the steps and rest one minute before completing the interval again.

Exercise	Sets	Reps	Resistance (%)
Stair Climb	3	-	90 - 100
Box Jump	3	5	90 - 100
Jump Rope	3	1 minutes	90 - 100
Push-up	3	25	90 - 100
Stair Descend	3	-	90 - 100
Rest Periods	Varies		

Workout 203
The Big Leagues

Class	Difficulty Level	Time
HIIT	Advanced	15 minutes

This is the only baseball / softball workout in the book; To perform this workout, begin by completing 5 all out sprints from home plate to first base. Rest at least 90 seconds between each sprint. Next, complete 4 sprints from first base to second base and 3 sprints from second base to third. All three of these sets of sprints are the same distance; the distances do not increase until the sprint from first to third base.

Exercise	Sets	Reps	Resistance (%)
Home to 1st Base Run	5	-	90 - 100
1st to 2nd Base	4	-	90 - 100
2nd to 3rd Base	3	-	90 - 100
1st to 3rd Base	2	-	90 - 100
All Four Bases	1	-	90 - 100
Rest Periods	60 – 90 seconds		

Workout 204
200 Reps

Class	Difficulty Level	Time
Mixed	Advanced	25 minutes

The 200 reps workout was created in celebration of the 200th workout. Here, you will complete four straight sets of 5 box jumps, rest, and then complete the circuit with the subsequent exercises. Finish with a two mile run.

Exercise	Sets	Reps	Resistance (%)
Box Jump	4	5	90 - 100
Push-up	3	15	90 - 100
Chin - Up	3	15	90 - 100
Cable Curl	3	15	90 - 100
Cable Press-down	3	15	90 - 100
2 Mile Run	1	-	-
Rest Periods	Varies		

Workout 205
The Redneck

Class	Difficulty Level	Time
Mixed	Advanced	25 minutes

This is a workout that you can do if you're tired of the gym but are still looking to get a good sweat. Start by marking off around 40 yards in a straight line through a field, and then find a muddy area of about the same length. Next, set up several logs preferably near a small hill. Begin the workout by pushing your four wheeler from the start to the end point of the 40 yards. Immediately run the mud 40 and then begin stacking one log that you previously set up.

Exercise	Sets	Reps	Resistance (%)
Four Wheeler Push	3	40 Yards	BW
Mud Run	3	40 Yards	BW
Wood Stack	3	1 minute	BW
Rest Periods	Varies		

Workout 206
Treadmill Sprint Walk

Class	Difficulty Level	Time
HIIT	Advanced	15 minutes

This is a quick hitting treadmill workout that will allow you to burn a significant amount of calories in a short amount of time. Additionally, performing sprints can help boost your oxygen debt for long after you finish, further increasing the amount of calories that you will burn. Exercising at a high intensity increases the amount of oxygen that our bodies need beyond what we are capable of bringing in during the exercise bout. This causes your body to bring in more oxygen post exercise, which leads to an increase in calories burned at rest (6).

Exercise	Sets	Reps	Resistance (%)
Sprint	8	15 seconds	BW
Jog	8	45 seconds	90
Rest Periods	-		

Workout 207
Push Sprint

Class	Difficulty Level	Time
HIIT	Advanced	10 minutes

Following a thorough warm-up, begin this workout with 40 push-ups followed immediately by a sprint at 85 – 90% intensity (perceived). Rest 20 seconds, and then complete 10 fewer push-ups than the previous set, followed immediately by a 2 lap run at 80% intensity. After the 2 lap run, complete 10 fewer push-ups followed by a 3 lap run at 70% intensity and then finish with 10 push-ups.

Exercise	Sets	Reps	Resistance (%)
Push-ups	1	40	BW
1 Lap Run	1	-	90
Push-ups	1	30	BW
2 Lap Run	1	-	80
Push-ups	1	20	BW
3 Lap Run	1	-	70
Push-ups	1	10	BW
Rest Periods	2 minutes		

Workout 208
Hangin HIIT

Class	Difficulty Level	Time
HIIT	Advanced	30 minutes

The first exercise in this high intensity workout is the dumbbell hang-clean. The optimal way to set this workout up is to grab a pair of dumbbells and take them over to a cable cross machine. Attach a rope attachment to the cable cross machine, and move it to the top setting. Perform the interval below with no rest between each exercise and only 30 seconds of rest between sets.

Exercise	Sets	Reps	Resistance (%)
Dumbbell Hang Clean	5	10	60
Pull-up	5	10	BW
Push-up	5	10	BW
Rope Cable Crunch	5	10	60
Rest Periods	60 seconds		

Workout 209
Sprint Crunch

Class	Difficulty Level	Time
HIIT	Advanced	15 minutes

This workout will have your abs completely exhausted by the time you finish, which won't be long. Begin with 100 crunches followed immediately by a 50 yard sprint. Next, complete sets of 80, 60, and 40 crunches with 50 yard sprints interspersed between sets. Be sure not to jerk the back of your head on the crunches, particularly as you fatigue in the middle and at the end of the workout. Use your abs to pull your upper body off the ground and toward your knees.

Exercise	Sets	Reps	Resistance (%)
Crunch	1	100	BW
Sprint	1	50 yds.	90 - 100
Crunch	1	80	BW
Sprint	1	50 yds.	90 - 100
Crunch	1	60	BW
Sprint	1	50 yds.	90 - 100
Crunch	1	50	BW
Sprint	1	50 yds.	90 - 100
Rest Periods		15 seconds	

Workout 210
HIITastic

Class	Difficulty Level	Time
HIIT	Advanced	30 minutes

This workout is not all that complicated from a programming standpoint, but it is quite difficult. Begin with a plank rotation, and hold a neutral plank, a right side plank, and a left side plank for 30 seconds each for 3 minutes, rotating between holds. Next, run one mile on a track, treadmill, or outside at a relatively fast pace; finish with another plank rotation.

Exercise	Sets	Reps	Resistance (%)
Plank Rotation	1	3 minutes	BW
1 Mile Run	1	-	BW
Plank Rotation	1	3 minutes	BW
Rest Periods		2 minutes	

Chapter 8

Chest and Triceps Workouts

The final three chapters in this book will feature combinations of previous workouts that have been adjusted for key factors such as fatigue and time. Combining large muscle groups with smaller muscle groups has long been accepted as a viable way to achieve muscle gaining goals. As stated earlier, one of the key reasons that this method works is that training larger muscle groups results in a greater hormone release, which may aid growth in all of the muscles being trained during that workout, including the smaller ones (10). In contrast, a drawback to training smaller muscle groups in the same workout as larger muscle groups is that these smaller muscles will be more fatigued following a large muscle group workout, and you will be unable to lift with as much intensity. Therefore, the best approach to training smaller muscle groups may be to strike a balance between days of training these muscles by themselves and days of training them after training a larger muscle group. A good warmup for the workouts in this section would include push-ups or a series of light bench presses.

Chest and Triceps: Power Workouts

Workout 211
Bodyweight Power

Class	Difficulty Level	Time
Power	Beginner	30 minutes

This workout is intended to help you develop power while only using your body weight as resistance. Begin with plyometric push-ups. Here, assume a push-up position and then perform the down portion of the push-up on a two second pace. Next, explosively press back up as quickly as possible. Complete three sets of 6 reps of all of the exercises in this manner with 90 seconds – 2 minutes of rest between sets.

Exercise	Sets	Reps	Resistance
Plyo Push-ups	3	6	BW
Band Push-ups	3	6	BW
Narrow Push-ups	3	8	BW
Band Triceps Extension	3	8	BW
Rest Periods		90 seconds - 2 minutes	

Workout 212
Bench Power

Class	Difficulty Level	Time
Power	Beginner	25 minutes

Bench Power is a great workout for developing power in your upper body, particularly in your chest, shoulders, and triceps. Begin with three sets of bench press and concentrate on exploding up with each rep. Next, narrow your grip to just inside shoulder width and perform three sets of 5 close-grip bench presses. Take at least 2 minutes of rest between sets and focus on keeping your elbows tight and upper back flat against the bench. Focus on breathing in during the eccentric portion of each rep and out on the concentric portion.

Exercise	Sets	Reps	Resistance (%)
Bench Press	3	5	70 - 75
Close Grip Bench Press	3	5	70 - 75
·iods			2 minutes

Workout 213
Bodyweight Power

Class	Difficulty Level	Time
Power	Intermediate	30 minutes

Begin this body-weight power workout with explosive dips, performing the eccentric phase at a slow, 4 second pace and the concentric portion of the lift as quickly and explosively as possible. Next, grab a medicine ball and place it on a clear spot on the floor. Assume a push-up position with one hand on the ball. As you push up explosively, roll the ball to the other hand and catch it with that hand as you descend toward the floor. Alternate between each hand for 6 total reps.

Exercise	Sets	Reps	Resistance (%)
Plyo Dips	3	5	BW
Med Ball Push-ups	3	6	BW
Plyo Push-ups	3	6	BW
Narrow Push-ups	3	8	BW
Triceps Extension	3	8	BW
Rest Periods		2 minutes	

Workout 214
Dumbbell Chest Tri

Class	Difficulty Level	Time
Power	Intermediate	30 minutes

This dumbbell workout is meant to help develop power throughout your upper body, particularly in your chest and triceps. Begin with three sets of 6 dumbbell bench presses followed by three sets of incline and three sets of decline dumbbell bench presses. Next, perform two sets of behind the head dumbbell triceps extensions with a single heavy dumbbell followed by unilateral dumbbell kickbacks.

Exercise	Sets	Reps	Resistance (%)
Dumbbell Bench Press	3	6	70 - 80
Incline Dumbbell Press	3	6	70 - 80
Decline Dumbbell Press	3	6	70 - 80
Dumbbell Triceps Ext.	2	8	70 - 80
Dumbbell Kick Back	2	8 (Each Arm)	70 - 80
Rest Periods		2 minutes	

Workout 215
Best Day Chest Day

Class	Difficulty Level	Time
Power	Advanced	30 minutes

This is an old fashion chest and triceps workout that only utilizes heavy, compound movements in order to help develop power in the upper body. Begin with three sets of 6 explosive bench presses followed by three sets of 8 dumbbell bench press reps. Next, move back to the bench press and complete three sets of 8 close grip bench presses, still using explosive reps. Finally, finish with weighted dips, using either a weight belt attached to a plate with a belt or a dumbbell between your feet.

Exercise	Sets	Reps	Resistance (%)
Bench Press	3	6	70 - 80
Dumbbell Bench Press	3	8	70 - 80
Close Grip Bench Press	3	8	70 – 80
Weighted Dips	3	10	10 – 45 lbs.
Rest Periods			2 minutes

Workout 216
Power Pro

Class	Difficulty Level	Time
Power	Advanced	30 minutes

This is a straightforward chest and triceps power workout that will be challenging to complete in 30 minutes, but it certainly can be done. Begin with three sets of 6 heavy dumbbell presses with 90 seconds of rest between sets. Next, move to close grip bench presses followed by incline machine presses, bodyweight dips, and flat dumbbell fly's.

Exercise	Sets	Reps	Resistance (%)
Dumbbell Bench Press	3	6	65 - 75
Close Grip Bench Press	3	6	65 - 75
Incline Machine Press	3	8	65 - 75
Bodyweight Dips	2	8	65 - 75
Flat Dumbbell Fly	2	8	65 - 75
Rest Periods			2 minutes

Chest and Triceps: Strength Workouts

Workout 217
Simple Strength

Class	Difficulty Level	Time
Strength	Beginner	25 minutes

This workout is just as straightforward as it looks: simply perform three sets of 5 reps on the bench press, narrow push-up, and dumbbell bench press. This is a relatively high volume of heavy weight so don't use this type of a workout perpetually. Be sure to use a spotter on each exercise and focus on form throughout the workout. Although this is a beginner workout, anyone can benefit from completing it if the use the correct resistance and rest period length.

Exercise	Sets	Reps	Resistance (%)
Bench Press	3	5	80 - 85
Narrow Push-up	3	5	BW
Dumbbell Bench Press	3	5	80 - 85
Rest Periods			90 - 120 seconds

Workout 218
Machinery

Class	Difficulty Level	Time
Strength	Beginner	25 minutes

This workout is all about the machines. Free weights are great for building strength, but for beginners, machines offer a desirable performance / safety ratio. Machines allow you to push a lot more weight without worrying about stabilizing it, which can help with building the neural connections you initially need to build strength. This program includes three versions of the chest press, along with one triceps specific exercise.

Exercise	Sets	Reps	Resistance (%)
Machine Chest Press	3	6	75 - 80
Machine Incline Press	3	6	75 - 80
Machine Decline Press	3	8	75 - 80
Machine Triceps Press down	3	10	75 - 80
Rest Periods			90 seconds

Workout 219
Incline Strong

Class	Difficulty Level	Time
Strength	Intermediate	30 minutes

If you're looking to mix it up a bit while building strength in your upper chest, triceps, and shoulders, this is an excellent choice for you. Begin by completing three straight sets of incline bench presses, followed by three sets of incline dumbbell presses, and three sets of incline close grip bench presses. Finish the workout with incline skull crushers using an EZ bar.

Exercise	Sets	Reps	Resistance (%)
Incline Bench Press	3	6	75 - 80
Incline Dumbbell Press	3	8	75 - 80
Close Grip Incline Press	3	8	75 - 80
Incline Skull Crusher	3	10	60
Rest Periods			60 - 90 seconds

Workout 220
Decline Strong

Class	Difficulty Level	Time
Strength	Intermediate	30 minutes

Begin this lower chest and triceps workout with three straight sets of 6 dumbbell decline presses. Next, make your way over to the smith machine and perform three sets of 6 decline smith presses. The reason to perform dumbbell presses before smith presses is that, even though you could likely press more weight overall on the smith machine, from a safety perspective, it is sometimes best to perform dynamic exercises that require a high amount of stabilization prior to performing machine-based exercises.

Exercise	Sets	Reps	Resistance (%)
Dumbbell Decline Bench Press	3	6	75 - 80
Smith Machine Decline Press	3	6	75 - 80
Bodyweight Dips	3	8	75 - 80
Cable Press-down	3	10	75 - 80
Rest Periods			60 - 90 seconds

Workout 221
Flat-out Strong

Class	Difficulty Level	Time
Strength	Advanced	30 minutes

This is one of those workouts that requires a beast-mode mindset. Begin with three heavy straight sets of bench presses followed by three sets each of dumbbell bench, close grip bench, and reverse bench, all on a flat bench. Make sure to use a spotter throughout this workout and to continue to focus on using proper form as the workout progresses. It is not advisable to perform pressing-only workouts continuously, as you may develop overuse injuries, but this is a great way to mix things up occasionally.

Exercise	Sets	Reps	Resistance (%)
Bench Press	3	6	75 - 80
Dumbbell Bench Press	3	6	75 - 80
Close Grip Bench Press	3	8	75 - 80
Reverse Bench Press	3	8	75 - 80
Rest Periods			90 seconds

Workout 222
Barbells

Class	Difficulty Level	Time
Strength	Advanced	30 minutes

Barbells are one of the most useful tools in the gym for helping people build strength. In short, if you want to get strong, you need to use barbells. Begin this workout with two sets of standard bench presses. Follow this up immediately with incline bench presses and then close grip bench presses. Next, perform a reverse grip bench press on a flat bench. This exercise will target your triceps and the upper portion of your pectoralis major and it is a great alternative to close grip incline bench presses.

Exercise	Sets	Reps	Resistance (%)
Bench Press	2	6	75-85
Incline Bench Press	2	6	75-85
Close Grip Bench Press	2	8	75-85
Reverse Bench Press	2	8	75-85
Decline Bench Press	2	8	75-85
Rest Periods			90 seconds

Chest and Triceps: Muscle Building Workouts

Workout 223
Smithed

Class	Difficulty Level	Time
Muscle Building	Beginner	30 minutes

This smith machine workout is great for a beginner who is looking to add muscle mass or for someone that is more advanced, but looking to mix things up a bit. Though it may look like it will take longer than 30 minutes, it can actually be completed rather quickly because each exercise takes place at the smith machine, which minimizes the setup time.

Exercise	Sets	Reps	Resistance (%)
Smith Bench Press	3	8 - 10	75 - 80
Smith Incline Press	3	8 - 10	75 - 80
Smith Decline Press	3	8 – 10	75 - 80
Smith Close Grip Press	3	8 - 10	75 - 80
Rest Periods			60 - 90 seconds

Workout 224
Max Machinery

Class	Difficulty Level	Time
Muscle Building	Beginner	25 minutes

Although there are many trainers out there who have denounced using machines for strength training, machines can and should play a role in most people's strength training programs. Machine exercises provide a great way to gain size because you can go heavy with short rest periods without having to worry about stabilizing the weight. Here, begin with three sets of 8 machine chest presses followed by straight sets of machine incline, decline, and triceps presses. Finish with triceps press-downs.

Exercise	Sets	Reps	Resistance (%)
Machine Flat Chest Press	2	8	75 - 80
Machine Incline Press	2	8	75 - 80
Machine Decline Press	2	8	75 - 80
Triceps Press Machine	3	10	75 - 80
Rope Triceps Press-down	3	12	70
Rest Periods			60 - 90 seconds

122

Workout 225
Beach Muscles

Class	Difficulty Level	Time
Muscle Building	Intermediate	30 minutes

This workout begins with dumbbell bench presses and then moves to a barbell incline press. Additionally, this workout, like many in this chapter, utilizes dips in order to place an emphasis on both the muscles of the chest and the triceps. Follow up the dips with cable crossovers and finish with rope cable press-downs. Superset the dips with the cable crossovers to add intensity to this workout and to decrease the workout time.

Exercise	Sets	Reps	Resistance (%)
Dumbbell Bench Press	3	8	80
Incline Bench Press	3	10	70
Dips	3	10	70
Cable Crossover	3	12	60
Rope Cable Press-down	3	12	60
Rest Periods			60 - 90 seconds

Workout 226
Dumbbells Only

Class	Difficulty Level	Time
Muscle Building	Intermediate	30 minutes

Begin with standard, straight set dumbbell bench presses followed by dumbbell incline and decline presses. Next, move on to overhead dumbbell extensions with one heavy dumbbell and then finish the workout with unilateral dumbbell kickbacks. This workout moves from predominately chest targeting exercises to predominately triceps targeting exercises. This is done to ensure that both safety and performance are maximized.

Exercise	Sets	Reps	Resistance (%)
Dumbbell Bench Press	3	8 - 10	75 - 80
Dumbbell Incline Press	3	8 - 10	75 - 80
Dumbbell Decline Press	3	8 – 10	75 - 80
Overhead Dumbbell Ext.	2	8 - 10	75 - 80
Dumbbell Kickback	2	12	60
Rest Periods			60 - 90 seconds

Workout 227
Functional Muscle Building

Class	Difficulty Level	Time
Muscle Building	Advanced	30 minutes

Performing the following functional moves while manipulating the intensity by varying the rep speed, volume, and rest periods, will help you gain muscle without traditional weight lifting. Begin this workout with weighted dips, using a weight belt and plate or a dumbbell between your feet. Next, perform three straight sets of 10 plyo push-ups, followed by three straight sets of 10 incline push-ups with your feet up on a box or bench. Finish with a suspension trainer chest fly, or a cable fly if you do not have access to a suspension trainer.

Exercise	Sets	Reps	Resistance (%)
Weighted Dips	3	10	75 - 80
Plyo Push-ups	3	10	75 - 80
Incline Push-ups	3	10	75 - 80
Suspension Chest Fly	3	10	BW
Rest Periods			60 seconds

Workout 228
The Beast

Class	Difficulty Level	Time
Muscle Building	Advanced	30 minutes

This is the ultimate 30 minute chest / triceps muscle building workout. Begin with three straight sets of dumbbell bench press. Next, complete two compound sets of incline barbell presses, incline cable fly's, and incline dumbbell presses back to back to back with no rest between sets. Finally, finish with four supersets of dips and rope cable press-downs.

Exercise	Sets	Reps	Resistance (%)
Dumbbell Bench Press	3	10	75 - 80
Incline Barbell Press	2	10	75 - 80
Incline Cable Fly	2	10	75 - 80
Incline Dumbbell Press	2	10	75 - 80
Dips	4	10	BW
Rope Cable Press-down	4	10	75 - 80
Rest Periods			60 seconds

Chest / Triceps: Endurance Workouts

Workout 229
Push-up Squared

Class	Difficulty Level	Time
Endurance	Beginner	25 minutes

Push-ups should be a staple of any upper-body muscular endurance workout. Perform these four push-up variations in back to back style, with no rest between sets. Once you've run through the full progression, rest 3 minutes and then begin again. This workout should toast your chest, shoulders, and triceps.

Exercise	Sets	Reps	Resistance
Push-ups	2	5 - 10	BW
Wide Push-ups	2	5 - 10	BW
Neutral Push-ups	2	5 - 10	BW
Close Push-ups	2	5 - 10	BW
Rest Periods	60 seconds		

Workout 230
Dip Challenge

Class	Difficulty Level	Time
Endurance	Beginner	15 minutes

This challenge is the simplest of all the challenges; the goal of this workout is to complete as many dips in a row as you can, wait two minutes, and then do it again. This will be a great measuring tool to see where you are; you may complete 2 dips or 20, but either way, it will give you a starting point.

Exercise	Sets	Reps	Resistance (%)
Bodyweight Dips	2	Max	BW
Rest Periods	2 minutes		

Workout 231
Double Dipping

Class	Difficulty Level	Time
Endurance	Intermediate	25 minutes

This unique endurance interval focuses primarily on the chest and triceps. Begin with weighted dips then move immediately to normal dips by removing the weight belt that you are using. Finish the interval with triceps-focused dips by lowering your legs underneath you and leaning a bit further back on the parallel bars. Perform three intervals of 10 reps on each dip variation with no rest between variations and 2 minutes of rest between intervals.

Exercise	Sets	Reps	Resistance (%)
Weighted Dip	3	10	10 – 25 lbs.
Normal Dip	3	10	BW
Triceps Dip	3	10	BW
Rest Periods		2 minutes	

Workout 232
Narrow Push-up Marathon

Class	Difficulty Level	Time
Endurance	Intermediate	10 minutes

Narrow push-ups target the interior portion of your chest as well as your triceps. The goal of this challenge is to complete 100 reps of narrow push-ups in as few sets as possible with only 20 seconds of rest between sets. For example, you may complete sets of 30, 20, 20, 15, 10, and 5. This would mean that you completed the challenge in six sets. Your goal for the next time you try this challenge is to complete it in six sets or fewer.

Exercise	Sets	Reps	Resistance (%)
Narrow Push-ups	-	100	BW
Rest Periods		20 seconds	

Workout 233
Run the Rack x 2

Class	Difficulty Level	Time
Endurance	Advanced	15 minutes

This is an endurance workout that can be treated as a single workout or as two burnouts following a longer workout. On each of these exercises, choose a weight that is essentially your 10RM and perform 10 reps with it. Next, immediately rack that and grab the weight that is 10 pounds lighter, and perform 10 reps with that weight. Immediately rack that weight and grab the weight that is 10 pounds lighter. Continue this until you have completed eight total sets of 10 reps.

Exercise	Sets	Reps	Resistance
Dumbbell Bench Press	8	10	Varies
Rope Cable Press-down	8	10	Varies
Rest Periods			2 minutes

Workout 234
Cross Press Superset

Class	Difficulty Level	Time
Endurance	Advanced	30 minutes

This workout is a series of supersets that combines various cable crossover angles with sets of narrow push-ups. Begin by completing three sets of 12 reps each of normal (high to low) cable cross-overs and three sets of 12 reps of narrow push-ups in superset fashion. Continue this trend throughout the rest of the workout, taking only 25 seconds to rest between each superset. This workout not only uses supersets, but it also uses the pre-exhaust technique on the chest muscles by hitting them with a single joint move immediately prior to a compound multi-joint exercise.

Exercise	Sets	Reps	Resistance (%)
High to Low Cable Cross	3	12	60 - 65
Narrow Push-up	3	12	60 - 65
Mid Cable Cross	3	12	60 - 65
Narrow Push-up	3	12	60 - 65
Low to High Cable Cross	3	12	60 - 65
Narrow Push-up	3	12	60 - 65
Rest Periods			25 seconds

Chest and Triceps: Mixed Workouts

Workout 235
Cable Chest Tri's

Class	Difficulty Level	Time
Mixed	Beginner	30 minutes

This workout is designed to be completed on a functional cable cross machine. Begin by adjusting the cables to about three fourth of the way to the top and perform heavy standing cable presses for three sets of 8. Next, keep the cables in the same position, but rather than performing a cable press, perform three sets of 10 cable crossovers. Next, switch the attachment from a D-handle to a rope and perform three sets of 12 rope press-downs. Finish with a straight bar reverse press-down for three sets of 12 reps.

Exercise	Sets	Reps	Resistance (%)
Cable Press	3	8	85
Cable Cross	3	10	80
Rope Cable Press-down	3	12	70
Reverse Press-down	3	12	60
Rest Periods			Varies

Workout 236
Chest to Tri

Class	Difficulty Level	Time
Mixed	Beginner	30 minutes

This is a great all-around workout that begins with two sets of 6 bench presses at roughly 85% of your 1RM. Use longer rest periods, up to 2 minutes, on this first exercise. As you progress through the workout, gradually shorten the rest periods so that towards the end of the workout you are resting only 30 – 45 seconds between sets.

Exercise	Sets	Reps	Resistance (%)
Bench Press	2	6	85
Close Grip Smith Press	2	8	80
Decline Dumbbell Press	2	10	70
Narrow Push-up	2	12	60
Rest Periods			Varies

Workout 237
Mixed Machine Madness

Class	Difficulty Level	Time
Mixed	Intermediate	30 minutes

This machine-only workout begins with a normal grip, plate-loaded chest press for three sets of 6 reps. Next, complete three sets of 10 reps of both plate-loaded incline and plate-loaded decline presses. Finish at the smith machine with three sets of 15 close grip bench presses. Rest periods should begin at around 2 minutes towards the beginning of the workout and taper down to shorter and shorter periods as the workout progresses.

Exercise	Sets	Reps	Resistance (%)
Plate Loaded Chest Press	3	6	85
Machine Incline Press	3	10	80
Machine Decline Press	3	10	70
Close Grip Smith Press	3	15	60
Rest Periods			Varies

Workout 238
Dumbbell Domination

Class	Difficulty Level	Time
Mixed	Intermediate	30 minutes

This workout begins with dumbbell presses and then moves to flat fly's. Next, the workout calls for two straight sets each of incline and decline presses followed by two triceps exercises: overhead dumbbell extensions and dual dumbbell skull crushers. In order for this workout to come in under 30 minutes, the set counts for each exercise are limited to two. However, if you have time to extend a few of the exercises to three sets, feel free to do so.

Exercise	Sets	Reps	Resistance (%)
Dumbbell Bench Press	2	6	85
Dumbbell Flat Fly	2	10	75
Dumbbell Incline Press	2	6	80
Dumbbell Decline Press	2	10	70
Overhead Dumbbell Extension	2	10	70
Rest Periods			2 minutes

Workout 239
All-Round Awesome

Class	Difficulty Level	Time
Mixed	Advanced	30 minutes

Begin this all-around chest workout with five heavy sets of 5 reps of dumbbell bench press to focus primarily on strength and perform these reps with a 2 seconds up and 2 seconds down pace. Next, perform four sets of 4 reps of bench presses with about 65% of your 1RM taking 4 seconds to lower the weight and less than 1 to press it back up. Use longer rest periods at the beginning and shorter rest periods towards the end.

Exercise	Sets	Reps	Resistance (%)
Dumbbell Bench Press	5	5	85
Bench Press	4	4	65
Incline Machine Press	2	8	70
Weighted Dips	2	12	60
Rope Cable Press-downs	2	15	50
Rest Periods			Varies

Workout 240
The Finisher

Class	Difficulty Level	Time
Mixed	Advanced	30 minutes

This is the last workout in the chest and triceps section, and therefore it is one of the most challenging. Begin with two sets of 6 heavy bench press reps, then move on to two sets of 8 incline and decline bench presses, followed by two sets of 10 dumbbell overhead extensions. Finish the workout with two sets of 12 rope press-downs followed by two sets of 15 cable crossovers.

Exercise	Sets	Reps	Resistance (%)
Bench Press	2	6	85
Incline Bench Press	2	8	75
Decline Bench Press	2	8	75
Dumbbell Overhead Ext.	2	10	60
Rope Press-down	2	12	50
Cable Crossover	2	15	50
Rest Periods			Varies

Chapter 9

Back and Biceps Workouts

As stated in the summary of Chapter 8, there are both advantages and disadvantages of training smaller muscle groups in the same workout as larger muscle groups. The following workouts almost all begin with larger back exercises, such as pull-ups, rows, or deadlifts, and finish with biceps exercises. The reason that the exercises are organized that way is that the biceps do much of the pulling during the back exercises and need to be fresh in order to optimize both safety and performance. Like many of the other chapters, beginner workouts will feature predominately body weight and cable work, while more advanced workouts include more complicated lifts. A good warmup for these workouts would include a series of chin-ups or reverse lat pull-downs, as well as cable rows and cable curls.

Back and Biceps: Power Workouts

Workout 241
Bodyweight Back Bi Power

Class	Difficulty Level	Time
Power	Beginner	30 minutes

There's no need for heavy weight on this workout. Begin with two sets of 5 reps of inverted suspension rows, lowering yourself slowly and exploding back up on each rep. Next, perform explosive neutral grip pull-ups for two sets of 5 reps, again with a slow eccentric, and explosive concentric rep scheme. Finally, shift the focus to the biceps by performing reverse inverted rows on a smith machine followed by suspension biceps curls.

Exercise	Sets	Reps	Resistance
Inverted Suspension Row	2	5	BW
Chin-up	2	5	BW
Inverted Reverse Smith Row	2	5	BW
Suspension Biceps Row	2	5	BW
Rest Periods			90 seconds

Workout 242
Power to the People

Class	Difficulty Level	Time
Power	Beginner	30 minutes

Part of the goal of this book is to show that there are nearly infinite variations to workouts and that you should never get bored with exercise. I want to drive that point home by throwing in a fill in the blank exercise as the last one in this workout. The workout is pretty self-explanatory until you get to the last exercise, which is "Your Favorite Curl." Simply insert your favorite biceps exercise into this slot and complete two sets of 8.

Exercise	Sets	Reps	Resistance (%)
Reverse Bent Row	2	5	70
Cable Row	2	8	70
Dumbbell Hammer Curl	2	8	60
Your Favorite Curl	2	8	60
Rest Periods			90 seconds

132

Workout 243
Explosive Pull

Class	Difficulty Level	Time
Power	Intermediate	30 minutes

Begin this workout with three sets of 5 bent over barbell rows. Perform the reps with a 3 – 4 second eccentric phase, and an explosive .5 – 1 second concentric phase. Next, complete three sets of 5 pull-ups with a neutral grip, using the same rep timing as you used on the first exercise. In order to largely target the biceps while still working the back muscles, the next exercise is a reverse cable curl with a straight bar attachment. Finally, finish the workout with three sets of 5 explosive chin-ups.

Exercise	Sets	Reps	Resistance (%)
Bent Row	3	5	70
Explosive Pull-up	3	5	BW
Reverse Cable Row	3	5	70
Explosive Chin-up	3	5	BW
Rest Periods			2 minutes

Workout 244
Power Pull / Chin

Class	Difficulty Level	Time
Power	Intermediate	25 minutes

One of the most functional moves that you can perform to develop power in your back is the pull-up with all of its variations. Begin this workout with weighted, wide grip pull-ups for three sets of 5 reps. Next, lose the weight and perform three sets of 5 explosive, neutral grip pull-ups. Finish this quick-hitting workout with three sets of 5 explosive chin-ups. Rest periods should last between 90 – 120 seconds between each set throughout the workout.

Exercise	Sets	Reps	Resistance (%)
Weighted Wide Pull-up	3	5	70
Explosive Neutral Pull-up	3	5	BW
Explosive Chin-up	3	5	BW
Rest Periods			2 minutes

Workout 245
Deadlift Power

Class	Difficulty Level	Time
Power	Advanced	30 minutes

This is a great exercise for developing strength and power. Begin this workout with four sets of 4 deadlifts using 70 – 75% of your 1RM. Next, move to wide grip pull-ups and perform four sets of 6 reps followed by four sets of 8 cable curls. This workout primarily targets the muscles of the back earlier in the workout and biceps later in the workout.

Exercise	Sets	Reps	Resistance (%)
Deadlift	4	4	85
Wide Pull-up	4	6	BW
Cable Curl	4	8	70
Rest Periods		90 – 120 seconds	

Workout 246
Back Bi Sumo

Class	Difficulty Level	Time
Power	Advanced	30 minutes

Sumo deadlifts are an excellent choice to help develop power in your glutes, hamstrings, lower back, and middle back. Begin this workout with five sets of 5 sumo deadlifts with 70% of your 1RM. Take 2 minutes of rest between sets. Next, perform five sets of 5 explosive bodyweight chin-ups. Finish the workout with four sets of 8 cable curls with your choice of a rope attachment or a straight bar attachment.

Exercise	Sets	Reps	Resistance (%)
Sumo	5	5	70
Chin-up	5	5	BW
Cable Curl	4	8	70
Rest Periods		90 seconds	

Back and Biceps: Strength Workouts

Workout 247
Cables

Class	Difficulty Level	Time
Strength	Beginner	20 minutes

The most important aspect of building strength is that you use a heavy enough load to stimulate muscle breakdown and protein synthesis (2). Most cable machines allow you to use enough weight on exercises like the lat pull-down and cable row so that you can actually build strength. A great aspect of cable exercises is that they often provide resistance through a greater range of motion and at different angles than do other machines or free weights.

Exercise	Sets	Reps	Resistance (%)
Lat Pull-down	2	5	90
Cable Row	2	6	85
Straight Arm Cable Pull	2	8	70
Reverse Cable Row	2	8	70
Straight bar Cable Curl	2	8	70
Reverse Cable Curl	2	8	70
Rest Periods			90 seconds

Workout 248
Machine Backed

Class	Difficulty Level	Time
Strength	Beginner	30 minutes

This is as straightforward as it looks: five sets of 5 reps of plate-loaded machine rows followed by five sets of 5 reps of plate-loaded machine biceps curls. While this is not a workout that you would want to complete every week, it will help you mix things up a bit in the gym and help to develop strength in your back and biceps.

Exercise	Sets	Reps	Resistance (%)
Machine Row	5	5	70 - 80
Biceps Machine Curl	5	5	70 - 80
Rest Periods			90 seconds

Workout 249
Dumbbell Back Bi Strength

Class	Difficulty Level	Time
Strength	Intermediate	30 minutes

This back and biceps strength workout is designed to be performed with dumbbells only. Begin with four sets of 4 dumbbell deadlifts using relatively heavy dumbbells. Be sure to keep your chest up, back flat, and head facing forward throughout this lift, as it can be difficult to maintain form while stabilizing the dumbbells. Next, move to single arm dumbbell rows for five sets of 5 reps followed by dumbbell hammer curls of two sets of 8 reps with each arm. After performing two sets of 8 normal dumbbell curls, finish with two sets of 8 reverse dumbbell curls.

Exercise	Sets	Reps	Resistance (%)
Dumbbell Deadlift	4	4	80
Single Arm Dumbbell Row	5	5	80
Dumbbell Hammer Curl	2	8	70
Dumbbell Curl	2	8	70
Reverse Dumbbell Curl	2	8	60
Rest Periods			Varies

Workout 250
Beastly

Class	Difficulty Level	Time
Strength	Intermediate	30 minutes

Weighted chin-ups are not only one of the more difficult exercises that you can do... they also make you look pretty beastly in the gym. Begin this workout with four sets of 5 weighted chin-ups. Next, complete three sets of 6 heavy lat pull-downs, followed by two sets of 8 heavy cable rows. Finish the workout with two sets of 8 EZ bar curls.

Exercise	Sets	Reps	Resistance (%)
Weighted Chin up	4	5	80
Lat Pull-down	3	6	80
Cable Row	2	8	70
EZ Bar Curl	2	8	60
Rest Periods			90 seconds

136

Workout 251
T Strong

Class	Difficulty Level	Time
Strength	Advanced	30 minutes

T-bar rows are a favorite of mine because stabilizing the T-bar can be easier than stabilizing on a barbell bent row. On this workout, begin with the T-bar row for four sets of 5 reps. I recommend loading on multiple 25 lb. plates rather than 45 lb. plates because the smaller plates allow you to pull the bar closer to your chest, which increases your range of motion and allows you to get a better squeeze at the top. Next, perform plate-loaded machine rows, followed by reverse grip smith machine bent over smith rows and smith machine drag curls.

Exercise	Sets	Reps	Resistance (%)
T-Bar Row	4	5	70
Machine Row	3	6	70
Reverse Smith Row	2	8	70
Smith Drag Curl	2	8	60
Rest Periods		90 seconds	

Workout 252
The Bull

Class	Difficulty Level	Time
Strength	Advanced	30 minutes

Begin this workout with a heavy T-bar row, which work the lats, traps, rhomboids, and biceps, and requires a great deal of stabilization from the legs and core. Next, move on to the lat pull-down and perform three sets of 6 reps. Follow this up with two sets of 8 cable rows and then two sets of 8 chin-ups. Finally, directly hit the biceps with two sets of 8 alternating dumbbell hammer curls.

Exercise	Sets	Reps	Resistance (%)
T-Bar Row	3	6	85
Lat Pull-down	3	6	80
Cable Row	2	8	70
Chin Up	2	8	60
Hammer Curl	2	8	70
Rest Periods		90 seconds	

Back and Biceps: Muscle Building Workouts

Workout 253
Back to the Machines

Class	Difficulty Level	Time
Muscle Building	Beginner	20 minutes

This is a quick-hitting 20 minute workout that is an excellent option if you are short on time and your gym offers these plate-loaded options. Begin with a plate-loaded pull-down, which is intended to simulate a pull-up. Next, move on to a heavy plate-loaded mid-row, followed by plate-loaded low rows; these exercises emphasize the muscles of the middle back. Finally, finish with a plate-loaded curl in order to directly target the biceps.

Exercise	Sets	Reps	Resistance (%)
Plate Loaded Pull-down	4	8 - 10	80
Plate Loaded Mid Row	4	8 - 10	80
Plate Loaded Low Row	4	8 - 10	80
Plate Loaded Biceps Curl	4	8 - 10	80
Rest Periods			60 seconds

Workout 254
Row Out

Class	Difficulty Level	Time
Muscle Building	Beginner	30 minutes

Pyramid set and rep schemes have long been utilized to help individuals gain size and strength. Perform the first set of the pyramid with a weight that only allows you to complete 6 reps. Subsequently lower the weight on the next set and then perform 8 reps. Do the same for the next set and complete 10 reps. Perform the first two exercises in this workout in that fashion but use by straight sets on the remaining three exercises.

Exercise	Sets	Reps	Resistance (%)
Lat Pull-down	3	6, 8, 10	85, 75, 65
Cable Row	3	6, 8, 10	85, 75, 65
Cable Curl	3	6, 8, 10	85, 75, 65
Rope Hammer Cable Curl	3	6, 8, 10	85, 75, 65
Rest Periods			60 - 90 seconds

Workout 255
Lat's and Bi's

Class	Difficulty Level	Time
Muscle Building	Intermediate	30 minutes

As if performing three sets of 10 wide grip pull-ups isn't difficult enough, this grueling workout asks you to follow that up with three sets of 10 neutral grip pull-ups. The transition from a back workout to a biceps workout begins with three sets of 10 chin-ups. From there, find an incline bench and grab a pair of light dumbbells. Lay back on the bench with the dumbbells to your sides. Using only your biceps and moving only at the elbow, curl the weight up under control. Slowly lower the weight back down and that's one rep.

Exercise	Sets	Reps	Resistance (%)
Wide Grip Pull-up	2	10	BW
Neutral Grip Pull-up	2	10	BW
Chin-up	2	10	BW
Dumbbell Incline Curl	3	10	75
Cable Curl	3	10	75
Rest Periods			90 seconds

Workout 256
Functionally Huge

Class	Difficulty Level	Time
Muscle Building	Intermediate	30 minutes

Begin this body-weight workout by completing two straight sets of 10 reps of medium – wide grip pull-ups. Next, move over to the suspension bands and complete an inverted suspension row, supersetted with chin-ups. Once you have completed two of these supersets, make your way to the smith machine and complete two sets of 10 reverse inverted smith rows.

Exercise	Sets	Reps	Resistance (%)
Pull-up	2	10	BW
TRX Row	2	10	BW
Chin-up	2	10	BW
TRX Curl	2	10	BW
Inverted Smith Row	2	10	BW
Rest Periods			60 seconds

Workout 257
8, 10, 12

Class	Difficulty Level	Time
Muscle Building	Advanced	30 minutes

The rep range that has been shown to elicit the greatest amount of muscle growth is 8 – 12 reps (2). Here, use the heavier rep scheme of 8 reps for the compound move: the bent row and the lightest rep scheme, 12 reps, for the exercises that require less stabilization. Perform the exercises below in straight set fashion with one minute of rest.

Exercise	Sets	Reps	Resistance (%)
Bent Row	2	8	80
Wide Pull-up	2	10	BW
Cable Row	2	12	60
EZ Bar Curl	2	8	75
Dumbbell Hammer Curl	2	10	70
Cable Curl	2	12	60
Rest Periods			60 seconds

Workout 258
Dumbbell Backed

Class	Difficulty Level	Time
Muscle Building	Advanced	30 minutes

The first exercise in this workout is dumbbell deadlifts because this move requires the most stabilization and brings the largest number of muscles into play. Try to use the same dumbbells for both of the first two exercises. Next, grab a slightly lighter pair of dumbbells and complete two sets of 10 bent rows followed by straight sets of dumbbell curls, dumbbell incline curls, and dumbbell hammer curls.

Exercise	Sets	Reps	Resistance (%)
Dumbbell Deadlift	2	10	70
Dumbbell Shrug	2	10	70
Dumbbell Row	2	10	70
Dumbbell Curl	2	10	70
Dumbbell Incline Curl	2	10	70
Dumbbell Hammer Curl	2	10	70
Rest Periods			90 seconds

Back and Biceps: Endurance Workouts

Workout 259
Dumbbell Endurance

Class	Difficulty Level	Time
Endurance	Beginner	20 minutes

Dumbbells are one of the best implements in the gym for building muscular endurance because they are so versatile. Use dumbbell exercises here to help you build muscular endurance in your back and biceps, beginning with single arm dumbbell rows. Next, move on to bent dumbbell fly's, a move that is typically used to work the rear deltoid of the shoulder but is also useful for hitting the muscles in the middle of the back. After finishing the back moves, perform two sets of 12 dumbbell hammer curls, followed by two sets of 15 dumbbell reverse curls.

Exercise	Sets	Reps	Resistance (%)
Single-Arm Dumbbell Row	2	12	65
Bent Dumbbell Fly	2	15	55
Dumbbell Hammer Curl	2	12	65
Dumbbell Reverse Curl	2	15	55
Rest Periods	60 - 90 seconds between exercises		

Workout 260
Chin-up Challenge

Class	Difficulty Level	Time
Endurance	Beginner	5 minutes

The chin-up challenge requires that you complete as many reps of chin-ups as you can in 5 minutes with only 20 seconds of rest between each set. If you can only complete 3 reps, keep your head up and try to get 4 the next time. This is a great test of both anaerobic and aerobic endurance and takes only 5 minutes after a warmup.

Exercise	Sets	Reps	Resistance (%)
Chin-up	Varies	Max	BW
Rest Periods	20 seconds		

141

Workout 261
Pull-up Curl

Class	Difficulty Level	Time
Endurance	Intermediate	10 minutes

This is a burnout that can be completed once at the end of a workout or multiple times for a single workout. Begin with the most pull-ups that you can do at once. Complete that number and then immediately drop and perform the same amount of reps of cable curls. Rest 15 – 20 seconds and then jump up and perform 2 fewer pull-ups than before, followed immediately by 2 fewer cable curls. Continue this for one more set and then rest.

Exercise	Sets	Reps	Resistance (%)
Pull-ups	1	10	BW
Cable Curls	1	10	60
Pull-ups	1	8	BW
Cable Curls	1	8	55
Pull-ups	1	6	BW
Cable Curls	1	6	50
Rest Periods		15 – 20 seconds	

Workout 262
Endure This

Class	Difficulty Level	Time
Endurance	Intermediate	30 minutes

Straightforward workouts are sometimes best; this is one of those times. This workout doesn't have any advanced intensity boosting techniques or any other tricks. Simply follow the formula below for a challenging muscular endurance back and biceps workout.

Exercise	Sets	Reps	Resistance (%)
Pull-up	2	12	BW
Plate Loaded Row	2	12	60
Chin-up	2	12	BW
Cable Row	2	12	60
EZ Bar Curl	2	12	60
Reverse Cable Curl	2	12	50
Rest Periods		60 - 90 seconds between exercises	

Workout 263
Hear the Pin Drop

Class	Difficulty Level	Time
Endurance	Advanced	10 minutes

Begin this workout with lat pull-downs; place the pin on a weight that will allow you to complete 8 reps, but no more than 8. Complete 8 reps and then immediately pull the pin and place it one spot up on the stack, slightly lightening the load. Complete 10 reps with this weight and then pull the pin and immediately complete 12 reps on the next lightest weight. Continue this to 15 and 20 reps. After finishing the lat pull-downs, rest 90 seconds and complete the cable rows and cable curls in the same manner.

Exercise	Sets	Reps	Resistance
Lat Pull-down	5	8,10,12,15,20	Varies
Cable Row	5	8,10,12,15,20	Varies
Cable Curl	5	8,10,12,15,20	Varies
Rest Periods	\multicolumn{3}{c}{90 seconds between exercises}		

Workout 264
Back All Day

Class	Difficulty Level	Time
Endurance	Advanced	10 minutes

Challenge yourself with this high rep back and biceps blaster. Begin with two sets of 12 pull-ups, taking 60 – 90 seconds of rest between sets. Next, move to the cable cross and complete two sets of 15 reps using a moderate weight. From there, complete two sets of 20 cable curls with light weight. Next, start over with two sets of 12 chin-ups followed by reverse grip rows and reverse grip cable curls.

Exercise	Sets	Reps	Resistance (%)
Pull-up	2	12	BW
Cable Row	2	15	60
Cable Curl	2	20	50
Chin-up	2	12	BW
Reverse Cable Row	2	15	60
Reverse Cable Curl	2	20	50
Rest Periods	60 - 90 seconds between exercises		

Back and Biceps: Mixed Workouts

Workout 265
Mixed Back Bi Machines

Class	Difficulty Level	Time
Mixed	Beginner	30 minutes

The 10, 12, 15 rep scheme below is ideal for developing a mix of hypertrophy and muscular endurance. Use a higher weight for eight rep sets and progressively lower the weight for twelve and fifteen rep sets. Use this rep and resistance scheme on each of the exercises below.

Exercise	Sets	Reps	Resistance
Plate Loaded Lat Pull	3	8, 12, 15	Varies
Plate Loaded Mid Row	3	8, 12, 15	Varies
Plate Loaded Low Row	3	8, 12, 15	Varies
Back Extension Machine	3	8, 12, 15	Varies
Plate Loaded Biceps Curl	3	8, 12, 15	Varies
Rest Periods	90 seconds between exercises		

Workout 266
Barred

Class	Difficulty Level	Time
Mixed	Beginner	20 minutes

Begin this workout with two sets of heavy deadlifts for 5 reps. Next, perform three sets of bent rows with moderate weight for 8 reps. Using the same bar as on the previous two exercises, perform four sets of 10 barbell shrugs to round out back training. Finish the workout by running the rack with fixed barbells. Begin with a heavier weighted fixed barbell and perform 8 – 10 reps. Rack that barbell and immediately grab the next lightest barbell and complete 8 – 10 more reps. Continue this until you have made your way through the entire rack.

Exercise	Sets	Reps	Resistance (%)
Deadlift	2	5	80 - 85
Bent Row	3	8	80 - 85
Barbell Shrug	4	10	70
Fixed Barbell Rack Run	Varies	Varies	Varies
Rest Periods	90 seconds between exercises		

Workout 267
BroMix

Class	Difficulty Level	Time
Mixed	Intermediate	20 minutes

This workout needs very little explanation. Every exercise is a straight set of the prescribed reps; for unilateral exercises such as the single arm and the dumbbell hammer curls complete the prescribed number of sets with each arm. Take between 60 – 90 seconds of rest between each set.

Exercise	Sets	Reps	Resistance (%)
Wide Grip Pull-up	3	6	BW
Single Arm Row	3	8	80
Back Extension	3	10	BW
EZ Bar Curl	3	12	70
Dumbbell Hammer Curl	3	15	60
Rest Periods		90 seconds between exercises	

Workout 268
The Ultimate Pull-up Workout

Class	Difficulty Level	Time
Mixed	Intermediate	30 minutes

This is the ultimate pull-up workout. Sure, you aren't doing as many pull-ups as you would in a pull-up challenge, but you are getting more of a variety than you will with any other pull-up workout in this book (and there are a lot of pull-up workouts in this book... that's because the pull-up is the best exercise known to man). Begin this workout with weighted, neutral grip pull-ups for three sets of 6 reps. Next, lose the weight belt and go wide for three sets of 8 reps. After the wide grips, move to a neutral, palms facing grip for three sets of 10 followed by three sets of 12 close-grip chin-ups. Take 60 – 90 seconds of rest between each set.

Exercise	Sets	Reps	Resistance (%)
Weighted Pull-up	3	6	70
Wide Pull-up	3	8	BW
Neutral Pull-up	3	10	BW
Chin-up	3	12	BW
Rest Periods		60 - 90 seconds between exercises	

Workout 269
From the Back to the Beach

Class	Difficulty Level	Time
Mixed	Advanced	30 minutes

Begin this workout with three sets of 5 reps of heavy deadlifts. Rest at least two minutes between each set of deadlifts. Next, move to reverse grip bent barbell rows with a moderate weight. It will be difficult to maintain proper form on the bent rows because the grip is reversed, and your legs are going to be fatigued from the deadlifts. Next, transition into biceps training by completing straight bar curls. Lastly, finish the workout with three sets of alternating dumbbell hammer curls.

Exercise	Sets	Reps	Resistance (%)
Deadlift	3	5	70 - 80
Reverse Bent Row	3	8	70 - 80
Straight Bar Curl	3	10	70
Dumbbell Hammer Curl	3	12	60
Rest Periods			Varies

Workout 270
Last Back Bi

Class	Difficulty Level	Time
Mixed	Advanced	20 minutes

Begin this workout with three sets of 6 weighted pull-ups with a 5, 10, or 25 pound plate attached to a weight belt with a chain. Next, grab a weight plate and make your way over to the back extension. Perform three sets of 8 back extensions; be sure to keep your head up, chest out, and back flat throughout this exercise, which can be difficult while using weight. Next, move onto a couple of a biceps moves: the dumbbell hammer curl and cable curls. Perform these exercises in three straight sets of 10 and 12 reps.

Exercise	Sets	Reps	Resistance (%)
Weighted Pull-ups	3	6	85
Weighted Back Ext.	3	8	80
Hammer Curl	3	10	70
Cable Curl	3	12	60
Rest Periods		90 seconds between exercises	

Chapter 10

Chest and Back Workouts

Most workouts in this book focus on a primary muscle group such as the chest, back, or shoulders and might include a few exercises from a smaller muscle group like the biceps or triceps. This is the standard way to build a workout but certainly not the only way. This chapter has 30 workouts that work both the chest and back in the same workout. Constructing a workout so that "push" and "pull" exercises are alternated throughout the workout can help to recruit more muscle fibers and help to allow muscle fibers to recover more between sets (2). This can lead to an ability to perform more sets and reps, which in turn can lead to greater increases in strength and hypertrophy. Here, chest exercises, which are primarily "push" exercises, are alternated with back exercises, which are all "pull" exercises. While you are performing the press exercises, your pull muscles have a longer chance to rest and recover, enabling you to come back to the next pull set stronger than you would if you completed several pull exercises in a row, and vice versa. The same goes for alternating actual sets between push and pull, which is indicated in several of the workouts in this chapter. A good warmup for these workouts could include a number of different exercises including push-ups, pull-ups chest presses, or machine rows.

Chest and Back: Power Workouts

Workout 271
Alternating Awesomeness

Class	Difficulty Level	Time
Power	Beginner	20 minutes

In this power workout you get to alternate between chest and back workouts. Perform each rep explosively but under control in order to stimulate the fast twitch muscle fibers in your chest and back. Be sure to keep your form in check, particularly on the cable rows and back extensions, as it can be easy to round your back on these exercises.

Exercise	Sets	Reps	Resistance (%)
Machine Chest Press	2	5	65 - 75
Cable Row	2	5	65 - 75
Incline Machine Press	2	6	65
Lat Pull-Down	2	6	65
Decline Machine Press	2	7	60
Back Extension	2	7	BW
Rest Periods	90 - 120 seconds between exercises		

Workout 272
Mr. Smith

Class	Difficulty Level	Time
Power	Beginner	30 minutes

Can you really design an entire workout around the smith machine? Absolutely. The smith machine is excellent for power training because it offers both flexibility and safety that free weights inherently lack. Perform each rep on the smith machine in an explosive but controlled manner. While the weight is anchored to tracks, it still is a good idea to use a spotter on this exercise.

Exercise	Sets	Reps	Resistance (%)
Smith Bench Press	2	5	85
Smith Incline Press	2	5	80
Smith Machine Row	2	5	75
Inverted Row on Smith	2	5	BW
Rest Periods	90 - 120 seconds between exercises		

Workout 273
Explosions

Class	Difficulty Level	Time
Power	Intermediate	20 minutes

These exercises can be performed in either straight sets or in a superset manner with no rest between the back exercise and the chest exercise. Whether you decide to perform these as straight sets or as supersets, be sure to take at least 90 seconds of rest between sets even if you don't feel like you need it.

Exercise	Sets	Reps	Resistance
Explosive Pull-up	3	5	BW
Explosive Dip	3	5	BW
Explosive inverted row	3	5	BW
Explosive Push – up	3	5	BW
Rest Periods		90 - 120 seconds between exercises	

Workout 274
Front 2 Back

Class	Difficulty Level	Time
Power	Intermediate	20 minutes

Begin this opposing muscle group workout with three sets of 5 moderately heavy bench press reps. Next, to get ready for the bent rows, remove some of the weight from the bar that you used for the bench press and straddle the bench facing towards the racked bar. Perform three sets of 5 reps using a moderately heavy weight. Subsequently, perform three sets of 8 dumbbell bench presses, still using only moderate weight, followed by three sets of 8 single-arm dumbbell rows. On each rep, lower the weight under control during the eccentric portion of the rep and explode back up on the concentric portion.

Exercise	Sets	Reps	Resistance (%)
Bench Press	3	5	70
Bent Row	3	5	70
Dumbbell Bench Press	3	8	70
One Arm Dumbbell Bent Row	3	8	70
Rest Periods		90 - 120 seconds between exercises	

Workout 275
Power Angles

Class	Difficulty Level	Time
Power	Advanced	30 minutes

Workouts like this are a great way to help you develop strength, power, and size. Use this workout to hit your chest and back from a variety of angles to help stimulate the greatest number of muscle fibers possible.

Exercise	Sets	Reps	Resistance (%)
Bench Press	2	5	70
Incline Bench Press	2	5	70
Decline Bench Press	2	5	70
Bent Barbell Row	2	5	70
Cable Row	2	5	70
Lat Pull-down	2	5	70
Rest Periods	90 seconds between exercises		

Workout 276
Last Power

Class	Difficulty Level	Time
Power	Advanced	30 minutes

Begin this workout with single arm dumbbell rows for three sets of 5 reps with each arm. To perform this move, place a moderately heavy dumbbell on the floor and stand on either side of it with your feet slightly wider than shoulder width. Bend over at your knees and hips, keeping your back flat, chest up, and head straight, and grab the dumbbell with one arm. To perform the lift, explode up by extending at your ankles, knees, and hips, while simultaneously rowing the dumbbell up to your side with your arm. Lower the dumbbell back down under control and then switch arms and perform the move again. Perform 5 reps with each arm.

Exercise	Sets	Reps	Resistance (%)
Unilateral Dumbbell Row	3	5	70
Explosive Smith Bench	3	5	70
Explosive Lat Pull-down	3	6	70
Flat Dumbbell Press	3	6	70
Rest Periods	90 - 120 seconds between exercises		

Chest and Back: Strength Workouts

Workout 277
Machinery Madness

Class	Difficulty Level	Time
Strength	Beginner	30 minutes

This plate-loaded workout is excellent for anyone looking to develop strength but limit their exposure to the risk of injury that comes with free weight exercises. That's not to say that you can't get hurt on a machine, you still can, but you don't have to worry about stabilizing the weight, which can lead to injury if you are unable to do so.

Exercise	Sets	Reps	Resistance (%)
Plate Loaded Chest Press	3	6 - 8	75 - 85
Plate Loaded Row	3	6 - 8	75 - 85
Plate Loaded Incline Press	3	6 - 8	70 - 80
Plate Loaded Pull-down	3	6 - 8	70 - 80
Rest Periods		90 seconds between exercises	

Workout 278
Cable Front to Back

Class	Difficulty Level	Time
Strength	Beginner	30 minutes

Cable crossover machines offer so much flexibility in terms of exercise selection that if you were to purchase one piece of equipment for a home gym, I would recommend one of these. You can often find a cable crossover in smaller gyms that only offer a limited amount of equipment; that's where a workout like this comes in handy. Perform all of these moves in a standing position, except for the lat pull-down. For the lat pull-down, sit with your legs facing the cable machine and attach two D handles to the pulleys. Pull the cables straight down in a lat pull-down motion.

Exercise	Sets	Reps	Resistance (%)
Cable Chest Press	3	6 - 8	75 - 85
Lat Pull down	3	6 - 8	75 - 85
Cable Fly	3	6 - 8	70 - 80
Cable Row	3	6 - 8	70 - 80
Rest Periods		90 seconds between exercises	

Workout 279
Rerun

Class	Difficulty Level	Time
Strength	Intermediate	20 minutes

Add some upper body mass to your frame with this heavy chest and back workout. Begin with the bench press for three sets of 6 reps, followed by the dumbbell bench version for three sets of 8 reps. Next, complete three sets of 6 bent rows with a straight bar, followed by three sets of 8 wide grip pull-ups.

Exercise	Sets	Reps	Resistance (%)
Bench Press	3	6	85
Dumbbell Bench Press	3	8	80
Bent Row	3	6	80
Wide Pull-up	3	8	BW
Rest Periods		90 seconds between exercises	

Workout 280
That Bar

Class	Difficulty Level	Time
Strength	Intermediate	20 minutes

It may not seem possible that this workout can be completed in 20 minutes, but it is designed so that you will be able to complete the entire workout using the same bench and bar, which significantly cuts down on time spent between lifts. Simply move from one workout to the next by adjusting the weight according to the exercise that you are about to perform. Use straight sets on this workout and be sure to grab a spotter for support.

Exercise	Sets	Reps	Resistance (%)
Bench Press	3	6	85
Bent Row	3	8	80
Close Grip Bench Press	3	6	80
Barbell Shrug	3	8	75
Rest Periods		90 seconds between exercises	

152

Workout 281
To the Limit

Class	Difficulty Level	Time
Strength	Advanced	30 minutes

Gaining strength is all about pushing yourself a little bit further than you did the last time. Do that here by attaching slightly more weight on the pull-ups, grabbing slightly heavier dumbbells on the bench press, using a little bit heavier weight on the T-bar, and dropping the pin a bit further on the cable rows than you normally would.

Exercise	Sets	Reps	Resistance (%)
Weighted Pull-ups	4	6	85
Dumbbell Bench Press	4	6	85
T-bar Row	4	8	80
Cable Crossover	4	8	80
Rest Periods	90 – 120 seconds between exercises		

Workout 282
Dumbbell Dude

Class	Difficulty Level	Time
Strength	Advanced	30 minutes

Begin this workout with standard dumbbell bench presses for four sets of 5 reps. Follow up the press with its antithesis: the bent dumbbell row. After the rows, move back to the flat bench for two sets of 8 dumbbell fly's and finish off the workout with two sets of 8 dumbbell pull-overs. To perform a dumbbell pull-over, grab a fairly heavy dumbbell and wrap your thumbs around the head of the dumbbell. Press the dumbbell straight over your chest and then slowly lower it in an arc behind your head. Keeping your arms straight, use your lats to pull the dumbbell back in front of your chest.

Exercise	Sets	Reps	Resistance (%)
Dumbbell Bench Press	4	5	80 - 85
Dumbbell Row	4	5	80 - 85
Dumbbell Fly	3	8	70 - 80
Dumbbell Pull-over	3	8	70 - 80
Rest Periods	90 – 120 seconds between exercises		

Chest and Back: Muscle Building Workouts

Workout 283
Front 2 Back Machinery

Class	Difficulty Level	Time
Muscle Building	Beginner	30 minutes

This workout is as simple as it looks: just three sets of 10 reps of each of these exercises. If you are a beginner, this workout will help you to establish coordination and a neural connection that will help you with future lifts. Although free weights offer more bang for your buck in the long run, machines are an excellent way to build confidence in the gym.

Exercise	Sets	Reps	Resistance (%)
Plate Loaded Chest Press	3	10	75
Plate Loaded Wide Press	3	10	75
Plate Loaded Pull-down	3	10	75
Plate Loaded Row	3	10	70
Rest Periods	60 - 90 seconds between exercises		

Workout 284
Bar Cable Body

Class	Difficulty Level	Time
Muscle Building	Beginner	30 minutes

This workout contains three chest exercises followed by three back exercises. Notice that the exercise order of the chest and back exercises mirror each other. The cable-based isolation exercises serve as a pre-exhaust to the compound bodyweight exercises, making them more difficult.

Exercise	Sets	Reps	Resistance (%)
Bench Press	2	10	75
Cable Fly	2	10	75
Push-up	2	10	70
Bent Row	2	10	70
Straight Arm Pull-down	2	10	70
Inverted Row	2	10	BW
Rest Periods	60 - 90 seconds between exercises		

Workout 285
Chest Press to Pull

Class	Difficulty Level	Time
Muscle Building	Intermediate	30 minutes

This workout is intended to be performed in superset fashion with little to no rest between the chest exercise and the back exercise. Perform five sets of 10 reps of dumbbell chest presses in conjunction with five sets of 10 reps of pull-ups. Begin the pull-up sets with wider grips and work to more narrow grips as you fatigue throughout the workout. Rest between 60 - 90 seconds between each superset but perform the pull-ups immediately following the dumbbell bench presses.

Exercise	Sets	Reps	Resistance (%)
Dumbbell Chest Press	5	10	75
Pull-ups	5	10	BW
Rest Periods		60 - 90 seconds between exercises	

Workout 286
Double Super-Sets

Class	Difficulty Level	Time
Muscle Building	Intermediate	30 minutes

This workout calls for two sets of supersets, one for chest and one for back. Set up the first superset by grabbing a light–moderate pair of dumbbells and placing them on either side of the front of a bench press that is loaded with about 70% of your 1RM. Perform 10 reps of bench press and then immediately after you rack the weight, grab the dumbbells and perform 10 reps of dumbbell fly's. Complete the second super-set in the same manner, performing the wide pull-ups immediately before the standing cable rows. Be sure to rest 90 seconds between each super-set and switch in dumbbell bench press for bench press if you do not have a spotter.

Exercise	Sets	Reps	Resistance (%)
Bench Press	3	10	70
Dumbbell Fly	3	10	60
Wide Pull-up	3	10	BW
Standing Cable Row	3	10	65
Rest Periods		90 seconds between exercises	

Workout 287
Functionally Big Chest and Back

Class	Difficulty Level	Time
Muscle Building	Advanced	30 minutes

Begin this difficult workout with a super-set of weighted pull-ups and weighted dips. Complete three super-sets of 10 reps of each exercise with no rest between the pull-ups and the dips and 90 seconds of rest between super-sets. Next, complete three super-sets of 10 reps of suspension trainer rows followed immediately by suspension trainer push-ups.

Exercise	Sets	Reps	Resistance (%)
Weighted Pull-up	3	10	70
Weighted Dip	3	10	70
Suspension Row	3	10	BW
Suspension Push-up	3	10	BW
Rest Periods		60 - 90 seconds between exercises	

Workout 288
Compound Interest

Class	Difficulty Level	Time
Muscle Building	Advanced	30 minutes

Begin this workout by setting up the first compound set. Grab a pair of heavy dumbbells, a pair of light dumbbells, and a light fixed barbell. A good rule of thumb is to use half of the weight that you use for heavy dumbbells for your light dumbbells and to grab a fixed barbell that weighs the same as one of the heavy dumbbells that you are going to use. Complete the back compound set in the same manner, using weights that allow you to complete 5 reps after you factor in fatigue.

Exercise	Sets	Reps	Resistance (%)
Dumbbell Bench Press	3	5	85
Dumbbell Fly	3	5	80
Barbell Bench Press	3	5	50
Wide Pull-up	3	5	BW
Cable Row	3	5	80
Straight Cable Pull-down	3	5	50
Rest Periods		60 - 90 seconds between exercises	

Chest and Back: Endurance Workouts

Workout 289
Push/Pull Challenge

Class	Difficulty Level	Time
Endurance	Beginner	30 minutes

This is a combination of two previous challenges in the book: the push-up challenge and the pull-up challenge. Here, feel free to perform either the pull-up or the push-up first or simply to alternate between the two (although it may be difficult to keep count that way). The goal is to complete 25 push-ups and 15 pull-ups in as few sets as possible with 30 seconds of rest between each set.

Exercise	Sets	Reps	Resistance
Push-ups	Varies	25	BW
Pull-ups	Varies	15	BW
Rest Periods	30 seconds between sets		

Workout 290
Big Pin's Droppin

Class	Difficulty Level	Time
Endurance	Beginner	25 minutes

Performing exercises in the 10 – 20 rep range enables you to build muscular endurance. Here, you will work through that entire range, decreasing the weight that you use as you increase the resistance. Begin this workout by completing one set of 10 reps of lat pull-downs with your 1RM. Rest one minute and complete another set, this time for 12 reps. Continue in this manner on the rest of the lat pull downs as well as on the cable crossover.

Exercise	Sets	Reps	Resistance
Lat Pull-down	5	10,12,15,18,20	Varies
Cable Cross	5	10,12,15,18,20	Varies
Rest Periods	5 seconds between sets		

Workout 291
Push Pull Variety

Class	Difficulty Level	Time
Endurance	Intermediate	20 minutes

This workout can be completed either in super-sets, with minimal rest between the back and chest exercises, or as straight sets. The exercises are ordered from the most to the least difficult so that you can finish the workout even after you are fatigued. Rest 30 – 60 seconds between sets and be sure to focus on your form throughout the workout.

Exercise	Sets	Reps	Resistance
Wide Grip Pull-ups	1	12	BW
Dips	1	12	BW
Neutral Pull-ups	1	12	BW
Incline Push-ups	1	12	BW
Narrow Pull-ups	1	12	BW
Push-ups	1	12	BW
Chin-ups	1	12	BW
Decline Push-ups	1	12	BW
Rest Periods	30 – 60 seconds between exercises		

Workout 292
Burpee to Pull-up

Class	Difficulty Level	Time
Endurance	Intermediate	30 minutes

Begin this workout underneath a cable cross pull-up bar or any other pull-up bar that has walk-through space. To perform the exercise, drop to the floor and swing your legs straight back while maneuvering your arms in front of you in a push-up position. Immediately and explosively press yourself up in a single motion and jump up in the air. When you reach the top of your jump, grab the pull-up bar and, without stopping momentum, complete a pull-up. That's one rep. Complete four sets of 10 – 15 reps.

Exercise	Sets	Reps	Resistance
Burpee to Pull-up	4	10 - 15	BW
Rest Periods	2 minutes between exercises		

Workout 293
Explosive Endurance

Class	Difficulty Level	Time
Endurance	Advanced	30 minutes

This is a hypertrophy/endurance workout. Begin by performing a set of 5 weighted dips. Once you have completed 5, strip off the weight and perform 5 explosive reps followed immediately by 5 normal reps. Complete three sets of these and then do the same for chin-ups. To complete the explosive reps, lower yourself down between the parallel bars on a 4 second count and, upon reaching the bottom portion of the rep immediately explode back up as quickly as possible while still maintaining proper form and control.

Exercise	Sets	Reps	Resistance (%)
Dips (weighted to explosive to normal)	3	15	50
Chin-ups (weighted to explosive to normal)	3	15	50
Rest Periods			20 seconds between sets

Workout 294
Stripped

Class	Difficulty Level	Time
Endurance	Advanced	30 minutes

If you've never used strip sets, you're totally missing out on one of the best ways to absolutely fry your muscles. The idea is basically the same as a pin drop burnout: load a barbell with several small plates, perhaps 10 lbs. and 5 lbs. then perform a set of 10 bench presses, strip one of the plates off of the end of the bar, and complete 10 more. Continue this until you are only lifting the bar. This should take between eight to ten total sets, depending on the weight that you start with. Rest up to 5 minutes and then do the same for bent-over rows.

Exercise	Sets	Reps	Resistance
Bench Press	10	10	Varies
Bent Row	10	10	Varies
Rest Periods			5 seconds between sets

Chest and Back: Mixed Workouts

Workout 295
Mixed Chest and Back Dumbbells

Class	Difficulty Level	Time
Mixed	Beginner	30 minutes

Perform each of the exercises in this workout in straight set fashion with 60 – 90 seconds of rest between each set, leaning toward longer rest periods on the first two exercises and shorter on the second two exercises. Additionally, use relatively heavy weight on the first two exercises but fairly light weight on the second two.

Exercise	Sets	Reps	Resistance (%)
Dumbbell Bench Press	4	6	85
Dumbbell Bent Row	4	6	85
Dumbbell Fly	4	12	60
Dumbbell Bent Raise	4	12	60
Rest Periods			Varies

Workout 296
Stairway to Hugeness

Class	Difficulty Level	Time
Mixed	Beginner	30 minutes

Begin this workout with two heavy sets of bench presses followed by plate-loaded chest presses and cable crossovers. After finishing the chest workouts, move to the back workouts and begin with the bent-over row. Be careful at this point to maintain proper form, as this exercise can be difficult to perform under any circumstance, especially when fatigued.

Exercise	Sets	Reps	Resistance (%)
Bench Press	2	6	85
Plate Loaded Press	3	8	80
Cable Crossover	4	10	70
Bent Row	2	6	80
Plate Loaded Pull-down	3	8	75
Straight Lat Pull-down	4	10	65
Rest Periods			20 seconds between sets

Workout 297
Mad Hatter

Class	Difficulty Level	Time
Mixed	Intermediate	30 minutes

This workout stair-steps up in reps and down in sets, load, and rest periods. This is done in order to push you through strength building, hypertrophy, and endurance periods in muscular development, all in one workout.

Exercise	Sets	Reps	Resistance (%)
Plate Loaded Chest Press	5	5	90
Incline Smith Press	3	8	80
Suspension Pushup	2	12	BW
Plate Loaded Row	5	5	80
Lat Pull-down	3	8	75
Suspension Row	2	12	BW
Rest Periods		60 - 120 seconds between sets	

Workout 298
Smoke Show

Class	Difficulty Level	Time
Mixed	Intermediate	30 Minutes

Begin this workout with heavy bench presses for only three sets of 5 reps with 85 - 90% of your 1RM. Next, complete the same number of sets and reps of pull-ups using a wide grip on the first set, a medium grip on the second, and a close grip on the third. Next, complete three sets of 10 cable crossovers followed by three sets of 10 cable rows. Finally, finish with three sets of 20 push-ups followed by three sets of 20 back extensions to work your lower back.

Exercise	Sets	Reps	Resistance (%)
Bench Press	3	5	85 - 90
Weighted Pull-up	3	5	85 - 90
Cable Crossover	3	10	70
Cable Rows	3	10	70
Push-ups	3	20	BW
Back Extensions	3	20	BW
Rest Periods		20 seconds between sets	

Workout 299
Top Tier

Class	Difficulty Level	Time
Mixed	Advanced	30 minutes

Perform the first two exercises in this workout as a super-set, followed by the second two exercises, and finally the last two. Rest two minutes between super-sets, but avoid rest as much as possible within each super-set.

Exercise	Sets	Reps	Resistance (%)
Dumbbell Bench Press	3	5	90
Flat Dumbbell Fly	3	10	60
Wide Grip Pull-ups	3	5	90
Straight Arm Pull-downs	3	10	60
Push-ups	2	12	BW
Cable Rows	2	12	50
Rest Periods	120 seconds between sets		

Workout 300
300th Workout

Class	Difficulty Level	Time
Mixed	Advanced	30 minutes

This is going to be one of the more challenging workouts in the book because it's the last. Perform the first four exercises as straight sets, taking 60 – 90 seconds of rest between sets. Perform the cable crossovers and push-ups as a super-set, as well as the cable rows and chin-ups.

Exercise	Sets	Reps	Resistance (%)
Bench Press	2	6	85 - 90
Explosive Pull-ups	2	6	85 - 90
Dumbbell Bench Press	3	10	70
Dumbbell Bent Row	3	10	70
Cable Cross	3	12	60
Push-up	3	12	BW
Cable Row	3	12	60
Chin-up	3	12	BW
Rest Periods	Varies		

Reference

1. ACSM News Release. (2013). Retrieved from: http://www.acsm.org/about-acsm/media-room/news-releases/2013/10/25/survey-predicts-top-20-fitness-trends-for-2014

2. Baechle, T. R., Earle, R. W., Wathen, D. (2008). Resistance Training. In Baechle, T. R. & Earle, R. W. (Eds.), *Essentials of Strength Training and Conditioning* (381 – 412). Champaign Illinois: Human Kinetics.

3. Bosco C., Tarkka I. & Komi PV. (1982). Effect of elastic energy and myoelectrical potentiation of triceps surae during stretch-shortening cycle exercise. *International Journal of Sports Medicine,* 3(3): 137-40.

4. Bosco, C., Tihanyi, J., Komi, P. V., Fekete, G. & Apor, P. (1983). Store and recoil of elastic energy in slow and fast types of human skeletal muscles. *Acta Physiologica Scandinavica,* 116(4): 343-349.

5. Bosco, C., Viitasalo, J.T., Komi, P.V., & Luhtanen, P. (2008). Combined effect of elastic energy and myoelectrical potentiation during stretch-shortening cycle exercise. *Acta Physiologica Scandinavica,* 114 (4): 557 – 565.

6. Cramer, J. T. (2008). Bioenergetics of Exercise and Training. In Baechle, T. R. & Earle, R. W. (Eds.), *Essentials of Strength Training and Conditioning* (22-39). Champaign Illinois: Human Kinetics.

7. Cronin, J., McNair,P. J., & Marshall, R.N. (2003). Force-Velocity Analysis of Strength –Training Techniques and Load: Implications for Training Strategy and Research. *Journal of Strength and Conditioning Research,* 17(1), 148–155.

8. Harman, E. (2008). Biomechanics of Resistance Exercise. In Baechle, T. R. & Earle, R. W. (Eds.), *Essentials of Strength Training and Conditioning* (65 – 91). Champaign Illinois: Human Kinetics.

9. Harman, E. & Garhammer, J. (2008). Administration, Scoring, and Interpretation of Selected Tests. In Baechle, T. R. & Earle, R. W. (Eds.), *Essentials of Strength Training and Conditioning* (250 – 273). Champaign Illinois: Human Kinetics.

10. Kraemer, W. J. (2008). Endocrine responses to resistance exercise. In Baechle, T. R. & Earle, R. W. (Eds.), *Essentials of Strength Training and Conditioning* (41 - 64). Champaign Illinois: Human Kinetics.

11. Ratamess, N., A. (2008). Adaptations to Anaerobic Training Programs. In Baechle, T. R. & Earle, R. W. (Eds.), *Essentials of Strength Training and Conditioning* (94-114). Champaign Illinois: Human Kinetics.